Ethical Theory and Pertinent Standards in Women's Reproductive Health

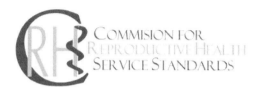

COMMISION FOR
REPRODUCTIVE HEALTH
SERVICE STANDARDS

Ethical Theory and Pertinent Standards in Women's Reproductive Health

The Foundational CRHSS Medical Ethics Manual

Rev. James R. Harden, M.Div

Carpenter's Son Publishing

Ethical Theory and Pertinent Standards in
Women's Reproductive Health:
The Foundational CRHSS Medical Ethics Manual
©2023 Rev. James R. Harden, M.Div

Published by Carpenter's Son Publishing, Franklin, Tennessee

Interior Design by Suzanne Lawing

Printed in the United States of America

Contents

Preamble

Medicine represents the intersection of the profound and practical, where science meets art. Because the clinician daily deals in the profound, he cannot afford to treat the practice of medicine as mundane. In Book 1 of *Metaphysics,* Aristotle noted the importance of practice and the even greater value of understanding the principles informing practice, saying, "We have said in the Ethics what the difference is between art and science and the other kindred faculties; but the point of our present discussion is this, that all men suppose what is called Wisdom to deal with the first causes and the principles of things . . . Clearly, then, Wisdom is knowledge about certain principles and causes."[1] It is the objective of this document to focus on the "first causes" and "principle" behind medicine and then to explore how those principles drive its day-to-day delivery.

---

1 Aristotle. *Metaphysics.* Trans. Ross WD. 1.1.7 [cited 11 Apr 2011]. Available from: http://classics.mit.edu/Aristotle/metaphysics.1.i.html. (981b27-30).

This understanding of principle is of ultimate importance in a society whose culture consists of differing views and interests. The American College of Physicians underscores this concern: "Today, the convergence of various forces—scientific advances, public education, the civil rights and consumer movements, the effects of law and economics on medicine, and the heterogeneity of our society—demands that physicians clearly articulate the ethical principles that guide their behavior, whether in clinical care, research, or teaching or as citizens."[2] It is not the intent of this document to be exhaustive in handling the relevant issues but only to describe them sufficiently enough to provide the reader context into the rich history and tradition of medical ethics—how the clinician has and should interact with society and his patients in the practice of the art.

Medicine mirrors society's beliefs about the ultimate nature of its subject, humanity. As such, and rightly so, the craft has been treasured with a reverence seldom paralleled throughout history. The aspiration to humanity's healer is noble and is perceived as noble precisely because of how humanity views itself. Humanity in general has articulated its own essential value in some of the most sublime documents of modern times such as the Declaration of Independence of the United

2 American College of Physicians. *Ethics Manual.* 4th ed. *Ann Intern Med.* 1998;128(7):577.

States; "We hold these truths to be self-evident, that all men are created equal . . ."[3]

The practice of medicine, like any other discipline, is informed by principles, and principles are informed by beliefs. Beliefs represent what Aristotle would call Wisdom, the "knowledge about certain principles and causes"[4] otherwise considered to be the reasons "why things are done" which in turn dictate "what things are done." Beliefs are typically informed by an overarching system of belief about the nature of things in general. This transcendent belief system determines principles or categories of behavior also known as "ethics" which in turn drive behavior or practice (see Figure 1 below).

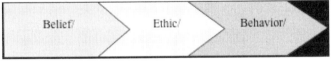

Figure 1

Medical ethics can be broken down into two categories of relationship; those between the doctor and society and those between the doctor and the patient. In both cases the doctor is always the noble servant and teacher, not an indentured servant. In both cases beliefs

3 *Declaration of Independence: A Transcription. National Archives,* U.S. National Archives and Records Administration, 8 June 2022, www. archives.gov/founding-docs/declaration-transcript.
4 Aristotle. *Metaphysics.* Trans. Ross. 1.1.7.

about those relationships drive how the doctor behaves or is expected to behave in any given circumstance.

Because we now find ourselves in a heterogeneous society, not just ethnically but also in terms of personal beliefs, moral dilemmas have increased. The moral crises that are faced by and often forced upon legislators, educators, judges, clergy, scientists, and medical clinicians are rooted in unavoidable complexity. This new reality creates tension within the field of medicine as colleagues differ on the ethical validity of research and treatment plans precisely because they differ in the beliefs impacting their understanding of the value and definition of humanity. Abortion, euthanasia, human stem cell research, infertility, even organ donation create ethical dilemmas within society not because of the issues themselves but because of the beliefs about the nature of humanity held by those providing the treatment or doing the research or writing the laws. Is a human defined by a utilitarian ethic in terms of what he can observably produce for society, by what conditions he can survive without assistance, or whether he has a sufficiently "good" quality of life? Or is a human life a physical representation of the image of God that therefore requires reverent protection? These basic beliefs or ideas are informed by what we will call transcendent authority (see Appendix A: Controlling Beliefs and the Idea of Transcendent Authority).

Transcendent authority informs those primary beliefs about the reason and nature of life itself. It is not the intention of this document to dispute or uphold the validity of one transcendent belief over another, but simply to note that they exist and, as such, inform how we treat each other. In fact it is because of the reality of heterogeneous controlling beliefs within culture and medicine that this document has been drafted.

This new reality requires clinicians to redouble their commitment to the historical principles of ethical engagement. In order to do this, they must first understand their own beliefs. It is when clinicians shut their eyes to their own controlling beliefs that they slip into the darkness of an intellectual arrogance, crippling their ability to understand and respect the differing controlling beliefs of their patients. When this happens, the clinician is in danger of compromising the patient's ability to make free and uncoerced decisions about their own treatment plans or those of their surrogates (those for whom they are responsible).

However one's controlling beliefs originate is inconsequential. The basic question each physician must ask him/herself is, "What is man?" The fact remains that the primary controlling belief that has informed the practice of medicine is the idea that each human being possesses intrinsic value. The practice of medicine must respect and dignify this intrinsic value. Medicine has done this by applying the traditional ethical principles of patient autonomy, beneficence, and non-maleficence to each patient relationship. These categorical imperatives, if removed, take with them the unconditional protection previously afforded every human, demeaning the role of physician to the level of veterinary medicine.

I. Traditional Categories of Medical Ethics

A. Doctor/Patient Relationship

Despite differences in social principles and cultural beliefs from generation to generation and even from doctor to patient as contemporaries there have been ethical commonalties to manage those differences that have been clarified in the passage of time through investigation or gross crimes against humanity. A core human principle understood by medicine and made clear in the Universal Declaration of Human Rights adopted by the United Nations in 1948 after the Nazi atrocities in WWII states in article 3 that "Everyone has the right to life, liberty, and security of person."[5] Nevertheless, the eventuality of ethical decision-making is something the clinician implicitly anticipates as he often holds that life and security of person in his very hands. The basic ethical concepts used to facilitate this important type of decision are common to traditional medicine and have been purveyed and promoted throughout the world in some form or fashion.

---

5 General Assembly of the United Nations. Universal Declaration of Human Rights. 1948, art. 3.

The following are ethical concepts having withstood the test of time guiding the clinician/patient relationship and will therefore be explored in the dynamics involved as medicine touches human reproduction.

1. Autonomy: Facilitating the patient's right to uncoerced choice or refusal of treatment.

2. Beneficence: A moral obligation to act primarily for the benefit of the patient.

3. Non-maleficence: First, do no harm. The physician's attempt to avoid any act or treatment plan that would harm the patient or violate the patient's trust.

Additional concepts such as informed consent, continuity of care, no conflict of interest, education, prevention, and confidentiality serve to clarify the three primary categories listed above and may overlap in support of each category. In recent years, some have attempted to redefine or place priority on one ethical concept over the others such as autonomy. But historically they have been viewed each as separate pillars holding up the sacred seat of medical standard of practice. This reality is underscored with the very existence of a medical ethics dilemma, since an ethical dilemma usually arises from tension or apparent conflict between two of the standard categories.

Communication is key to an ethical clinician/patient relationship, for all three of the primary ethical concepts in medicine depend upon it. Morris Abram, former Chairman of the President's Commission for the Study of Ethical Problems in Medicine and Biomedical and Behavioral Research states, ". . . the Commission sees 'informed consent' as an ethical obligation that involves a process of shared decision-making based upon the mutual respect and participation of patients and health professionals. Only through improved communication can we establish a firm footing for the trust that patients place in those who provide their health care."[6] One of many reasons why communication in the clinician/patient relationship is important is that it improves patient health. Studies have shown that the best patient outcomes occur in an environment of intentional clinician/patient communication: "Most of the studies reviewed demonstrated a correlation between effective physician-patient communication and improved patient health outcomes."[7] To expect that the patient is educated enough about their own medical condition or has the emotional wherewithal to reason through to a

---

6 Abram, Morris B. (Chairman, President's Commission for the Study of Ethical Problems in Medicine and Biomedical and Behavioral Research). Letter to: The President. 21 Oct 1982 [cited 9 Sep 2011]. 1 leaf. Printed in: Making Health Care Decisions: The Ethical and Legal Implications of Informed Consent in the Patient-Practitioner Relationship. Vol. 1. Washington: GPO; 1982.

7 Stewart MA. Effective physician-patient communication and health outcomes: A review. *Can Med Assoc J.* 1995;152(9):1423.

personally consistent treatment option is to miss the role of doctor as active educator.

The area of women's reproductive health poses a unique and ongoing ethical challenge where pregnancy is concerned. The reason for this is the fact that obstetricians are trained to deal with the complexity of a two-patient scenario when managing prenatal patients: the mother and her prenatal child. When there are health issues with the mother, treatment scenarios will likely impact the child and vice versa. In normal obstetrical circumstances where a healthy child is actually the mother's desired outcome, there is a presumption toward the life of the child by the physician. Some would say that this presumption is directly related to the subjective goal of the mother to have a healthy child. If that is true, it would dictate treatment options designed to optimize the health of two patients: mother and child.

However, in the context of women's reproductive health as it relates to unplanned pregnancy, it is often presumed that the goal of the patient is the opposite of a full-term pregnancy resulting in a healthy baby. Therefore, the subjective presumed goal of the patient as interpreted by the physician is pregnancy termination, thereby muting the two-patient issue of surrogacy typically handled by obstetricians: mother on behalf of prenatal child. This allows the physician to define the separation of the child from the mother for the purpose of fetal demise solely as the treatment of the mother. This presumption implies a patient service standard that is particular or subjective to the patient without taking into consideration the patient's actual perspective regarding religious beliefs, values, and goals. Simply put, the issue of surrogacy is rarely considered if the patient simply presents with positive pregnancy and requests an abortion. In fact, a 2004 study published in the *Medical Science Monitor* noted 84% of the American sample of women who had abortions said that they did not receive adequate counseling before receiving an abortion. Additionally, 64% felt pressured by others.[8] It is precisely the issue of whether or not surrogacy exists that causes abortion to remain a hot-button issue.

Moving toward a comprehensive, non-manipulative, clinician-led communication as an ethical non-negotiable would serve to abate much of the ethical difficulties; such communication provides the framework for the three traditional categories of an ethical clinician/patient relationship.

1. Autonomy

In recent years, the concept of patient autonomy has come to mean very different things to different people and has enjoyed inflated emphasis in ethics education

---

8 Rue VM, Coleman PK, Rue JJ, Reardon DC. Induced abortion and traumatic stress: A preliminary comparison of American and Russian women. *Med Science Monitor.* 2004;10(10):SR5-16.

and discussions. All of the other ethical principles—non-maleficence, beneficence, distributive justice, etc.—are presented as being secondary to and trumped by respect for autonomy. Physicians are encouraged to be more circumspect. This "respect for patient autonomy" as a mandate to facilitate any "legal" choice a patient may make without appropriate medical consultation may actually constitute an affront to the patient's self-determination—the very opposite of the concept of true patient autonomy.

This is particularly true in the area of reproductive health and at the end of life. This view of the ethical category autonomy lacks strength precisely because it represents the idea of ethical relativism and places the ethical principles of doing no harm and acting in the best interest of the patient as at least secondary ideas to the shallow notion of "whatever the patient wants," ultimately relegating medicine to just another consumer service degrading not only the patient but also the profession of medicine itself.

Happily, the classical notion of patient autonomy is a much more comprehensive idea and is connected to how a clinician empowers a patient's freedom by insulating that patient from coercive pressure and by providing all the information about her condition and treatment options.

Autonomous choice is meaningless unless the patient is empowered, educated, and informed. To make a truly informed decision, there are several aspects that point to a decision that is autonomous. Some of those indicators are that she is fully aware of her physiological and psychological condition; her decision is uncoerced and consistent with her personal beliefs; her decision is considered in the larger context of her future health and reproductive health goals; her options are carefully laid out, including the costs and potential side-effects; she is educated about the nature and physiology of fetal development; etc. Not only must the physician ensure that information is not manipulated when being delivered to the patient but also must ensure that no information is omitted. Justification of the omission of information for therapeutic reasons must be used sparingly if at all.

The essence of patient autonomy is derived from the transcendent belief both in the intrinsic value of a human life and that which in many ways reveals its value: self-determination. The ability for a human being to act as a free moral agent is a crucial belief in the practice of medicine without which even the practice of medicine itself would be compromised (see the concept of Clinician Right of Conscience in The Doctor/Society Relationship).

a) Self-Determination and Dignity

The notion of patient autonomy carries with it the basic presupposition of the dignity of all human beings. Humans desiring to be healthy are the "first cause" of medicine. The simple existence of medicine presupposes that patients have chosen to be served. Without the principle of patient autonomy medicine would not exist; and if it did exist, it would do so in a tyrannical environment. For medicine to serve a patient, that patient or surrogate must first consent to be served. For a patient to be served, the education and treatment offered by the clinician must be characterized by a mutual respect for the nature of humanity as represented in the form of a single human being. This could also be described as dignity.

Principles of Biomedical Ethics describes autonomy as "[encompassing], at a minimum, self-rule that is free from both controlling interference by others and from certain limitations such as an inadequate understanding that prevents meaningful choice."[9] Without a fundamental commitment to autonomy, a patient would be controlled and coerced by another human being, in this case, a doctor, who may hold very different ideas and beliefs about the nature of human life in general and how a patient in particular should then be treated. This disregard for the dignity of another human being is inconsistent with medicine despite the best intentions of a clinician.

9 Beauchamp TL, Childress JF. *Principles of Biomedical Ethics*. 6th ed. New York: Oxford University Press; 2009:99.

Because one cannot empirically confirm or deny the veracity of any particular belief or belief system, and because everyone holds to a belief or belief system that interprets the value and meaning of human life, the most conservative approach a medical clinician should default to is the belief that holds humanity in the highest regard. To illustrate, consider one medical clinician who practices according to a belief that a human being is simply a compilation of biochemical reactions with no intrinsic value and a second clinician operating under the belief that a human being represents God Himself. From which clinician could one reasonably expect to receive the best care? Which clinician would be more inclined toward active communication with the patient? Which clinician would be more likely to support the patient's autonomous decision-making ability?

Certainly the medical clinician should believe as their conscience dictates. However, ethical medicine requires that a clinician practice according to the belief which holds to the highest view of humanity rather than any view that reduces the dignity of a human life.

b) Informed Consent: No Information Manipulation

Theory

Patient autonomy is primarily supported by the notion of informed consent: free assent to a treatment option with comprehensive understanding. The idea is to insure that a patient's autonomy is maintained and that prevention and treatment decisions are free from controlling interference, thereby respecting the patient's dignity. Additionally it serves to insulate patients from any coercive pressure to make a decision inconsistent with their person and life goals. The National Abortion Federation states that "The goal of informed consent is to assure that the patient's decision is voluntary and informed."[10]

There are three generally accepted standards for understanding the appropriate ethical bounds of informed consent in the United States: (1) the particular (subjective patient) standard, (2) the materiality (reasonable patient) standard, and (3) the professional community (reasonable physician) standard.

The subjective patient standard requires information to be provided to the patient based on the particular circumstances and conditions of that patient. As it is extremely difficult for courts to establish informed consent under this standard in the case of alleged medical malpractice, state governments have favored either the materiality or professional community standards.

The materiality standard (e.g., reasonable patient standard) expects that medical clinicians present all information that a reasonable patient would consider

---

10 National Abortion Federation. 2011 Clinical Policy Guidelines. Washington: National Abortion Federation; 2011:3.

"material" to the decision-making process. The state of Utah, among others, adopts this standard, declaring that a failure to obtain informed consent has occurred when "a reasonable, prudent person in the patient's position would not have consented to the health care rendered after having been fully informed as to all facts relevant to the decision to give consent."[11]

The professional community standard, on the other hand, holds the clinician accountable to what other reasonable physicians would do in the same circumstances. The 2011 Florida Statute accepts this standard: "The action of the [physician] in obtaining the consent of the patient or another person authorized to give consent for the patient was in accordance with an accepted standard of medical practice among members of the medical profession with similar training and experience in the same or similar medical community."[12]

While there are significant variations in the way these standards view proof of informed consent, all three point to categories of information which must be communicated within the clinician/patient relation-

---

11 Utah Code 78B-3-406.1(f). Chapter 3, 2008 General Session; 2008 [cited 31 Oct 2011]. Available from: http://le.utah.gov/Documents/code_const.htm.

12 2011 Florida Statutes 766.103.3(a)1. Florida Medical Consent Law; 2011 [cited 31 Oct 2011]. Available from: http://www.leg.state.fl.us/statutes/.

ship: patient condition, patient values and goals, and treatment options. Without active communication between the clinician and the patient around these three topics, no standard judges that the process of informed consent is complete, and a clinician treating under such conditions violates medical ethics and is liable for medical malpractice.

The idea of informed consent is not simply a passive one degraded to simply signing a legal document of permission stating that she is of legal standing and has made a decision of her own volition. Unfortunately, informed consent documents in many instances serve as a replacement of active clinician/patient communication, whereby the clinician actively engages the patient in an open, confidential, and comprehensive exchange of information from her rights to the clinician's responsibilities so that the patient has complete understanding before a course of treatment is recommended.

This exchange of information around patient condition toward informed consent includes "the nature of the diagnosis,"[13] with any relevant diagnostic test information. Withholding such information is a serious affront to a patient's self-determination and autonomy,

13 Wear, S. Ethics Committee Core Curriculum: Informed Consent. UB Center for Clinical Ethics and Humanities in Health Care, University of Buffalo; 2006 [cited 31 Oct 2011]. Available from: http://wings. buffalo.edu/bioethics/man-infc.html

and the use therapeutic privilege to do so "can only be justified in exceptional circumstances"[14] (see Informed Consent: Education as No Information Omission for further discussion on justifications for non-disclosure). This discussion also includes an attempt by the clinician to understand the patient's personal, social, and emotional circumstances for the purpose of insulating her decision-making autonomy from external and coercive pressure. As the Pertinent Standards section indicates, this is done through access to the clinician with any questions the patient may have about her options after the initial consultation, as well as access to community resources to address and possibly remove any coercive pressures she may be facing. In so doing she can make a decision that respects her dignity and her controlling beliefs, while at the same time protecting her from being victimized by any contrary interests or beliefs held by others, including the clinician (see No Conflict of Interest).

In the context of women's reproductive health and specifically unintended pregnancy, pressure or coercion exists by the very nature of the life-changing circumstance of pregnancy. Pressure on a woman toward a specific outcome (i.e., pregnancy termination, full term, etc.) from people in her life such as parents, a boy-

---

14 van den Heever P. Pleading the defence of therapeutic privilege. *S Afr Med J.* 2005;95(6):421.

friend, etc., reveals the fact that almost every instance of unplanned pregnancy represents its own unique ethical dilemma that must be adequately addressed by the medical clinician through active communication.

A study conducted by the Guttmacher Institute confirms this reality, stating, "The decision to have an abortion is typically motivated by multiple, diverse, and interrelated reasons. The themes of responsibility to others and resource limitations, such as financial constraints and lack of partner support, recurred throughout the study."[15] This means that often the very consideration of abortion represents a symptom of a coercive set of circumstances which can only be addressed by a clinician committed to ethical medicine.

Furthermore, "When the patient's beliefs—religious, cultural, or otherwise—run counter to medical recommendations, the provider is obliged to try to understand clearly the beliefs and viewpoints of the patient."[16] Beauchamp and Childress add that "Respect for autonomy requires much more than avoiding deception and coercion. It requires an attempt to instill relevant understanding and to avoid many forms of manip-

---

15 Finer LB, Frohwirth LF, Dauphinee LA, Singh S, Moore AM. Guttmacher Institute. Reasons U.S. women have abortions: Quantitative and qualitative perspectives. *Perspect Sex Reprod Health.* 2005; 37(3):110.

16 American College of Physicians, *Ethics Manual,* 578.

ulation."[17] If the clinician does not know the patient's values, it is essential that he ask. This requires a level of communication that can only be facilitated by the clinician himself as well as a level of understanding by the clinician about his own beliefs to discern how they may be different than the patient's.

When a mutual understanding of the condition of the whole patient and her beliefs, values, and goals has been reached, the clinician must then present recommended treatment options and any existing alternative methods. Discussion of all potential treatments, including non-treatment, must include the general nature and description of each treatment, their relative risks, and prospects of success. Only then can informed consent—the patient's free assent to a treatment option with comprehensive understanding—be said to have successfully and ethically been attained.

The redefinition or violation of the traditional understanding of informed consent generates a litany of ethical problems. For example, for an abortion practice to market direct access to surgical or medical procedures disregards the idea of true informed consent especially if the clinician refuses to engage an open, two-way conversation as a matter of protocol. This is done by educating himself as to the patient's circum-

---

17 Beauchamp, Childress. *Principles of Biomedical Ethics*, 99.

stances and beliefs and educating the patient with respect to treatment options consistent with her beliefs and reproductive health goals. Generally speaking, specialized medical care advertising should be used with utmost discretion and caution (see the recommended Advertising policy in Pertinent Standards).

Medical advertising should align with basic medical ethics, rooted in education, focusing on prevention by encouraging the least invasive options first through medical consultation. Advertising a particular treatment outside the bounds of continuity of care could easily represent a conflict of interest and implicitly violate a patient's autonomy by taking advantage of an already coercive situation—unless the specialist doing the advertising reinforces proper expectations for informed decision-making and access to services. Medical specialist advertising when the service excludes the primary clinician/patient relationship could easily place the interests of the specialist clinician first, thereby violating the patient's autonomy, and, as such, represents egregious ethical error.

Pertinent Standards

(a) Patient Acquisition

Advertising
Policy stating that all advertising is educational in nature and attempts to encourage patient autonomy and continuity of care.

Explanation: Advertising encourages the patient to consider all less invasive treatment options with a medical clinician.

All advertising and scheduling sets the expectation that the patient will be provided with appropriate medical diagnostics and a complete options presentation.

The initial patient call is not simply scheduling. It contextualizes services and sets expectations.

Examples: Appendix II.B.1: Helpline Script,

Appendices II.B.2, II.B.3, and the Highland Hospital Bariatric Surgery website contain contextualized advertising examples.

Policy stating that for invasive, elective, procedures, the clinician must attempt to attain as much information about patient health history, socioeconomic background, and emotional state as possible.

Explanation: A specialist will request that a patient brings her health history with her to her first visit.

(b) Service

Policy stating that the clinician will establish a non-coercive environment by exploring with the patient all areas of influence that could coerce her choice.

Explanation:

Life situation: Any non-relational (material) influences, including educational, economic, geographic, etc.

Beliefs: Beliefs and values of the patient relative to the nature of human life, surrogacy, family, and religion which could impact treatment option recommendations.

Social pressures: Beliefs and values of the physician which may be at odds with those of the patient. The clinician communicates whether or not he/she will provide certain treatment options and why.

Pressure from counselors, nurses, parents, friends, the father of the baby, etc., toward any particular treatment option.

Examples: Appendices II.B.4: Patient Intake Form, II.B.5: Personalized Solutions Assessment

Policy stating that clinician must verify that patient is of bona fide legal standing to make her own medical decisions, including age and mental health.

Policy stating that a written patient bill of rights is provided to each patient, and is reviewed by the clinician with the patient.

Explanation: The clinician conveys the patient's rights and responsibilities to the patient both in writing and verbally to help ensure understanding.

Example: Appendix II.B.6 Patient Bill of Rights

Policy stating that the clinician engages with the patient in a thorough co-discovery process for diagnosing the physical condition of the patient.

Explanation: The clinician avoids moral entrapment, especially entrapment through withholding information (i.e., results of a pregnancy test) in order to convey an agenda to a captive audience.

The clinician avoids coercion, especially by leveraging all the diagnostic tools at their disposal to determine patient condition at initial visit, irrespective of Last Menstrual Period (LMP).

All data gleaned from diagnostic tests must be presented and explained to the patient, including sounds, images, etc.

Policy stating that written patient approval is required for any procedure (e.g., medical intervention), reviewed verbally to highlight any potential risks and side-effects, however remote, and the probability of success.

Example: Appendix II.B.8: Abortion Information Brochure, a sample review of the risks and side effects of abortion procedures.

(c) Follow-up

Policy stating that the patient is given access to contact the clinician with any issues or concerns while contemplating treatment options or after treatment is provided.

Policy stating that the clinician is to supply the patient with access to community support to address any obstacles to treatment.

Explanation: The patient is given access to community resources to help address coercive elements influencing her autonomous treatment decision. The clinician helps the patient develop a communication plan to appropriate people including her primary care physician, parents, boyfriend, community support, etc.

Example: Appendix II.B.5: Personalized Solutions Assessment

c) Informed Consent: Education as No Information Omission

Theory

Patient education represents the commitment of the physician to facilitate the co-discovery process between the clinician and the patient. This includes a commitment by the clinician to set the expectation that the patient will be provided with not only appropriate medical diagnostics and a thorough presentation of treatment options but also that the appropriate steps are taken by the clinician to understand the patient's context both medically and socially with sufficient time to consider her options. This exchange of information amounts to a co-discovery into a patient's whole condition with her clinician.

To clarify the point that education is the active responsibility of the clinician and is key in maintaining patient autonomy, the President's Commission states, "The health professional's expert knowledge, focused through the particular diagnosis and prognosis for the patient, usually confers on [the health professional] the natural role of leader and initiator in building this shared understanding."[18] The President's Commission goes on to say that "therapeutic privilege has been vastly overused as an excuse for not informing patients of facts they are entitled to know."[19]

By virtue of the nature of the clinician/patient relationship, the patient cannot be expected to know and understand what questions to ask, say nothing of whether or not certain treatment options will be consistent with her beliefs. Therefore, the clinician, under the ethical concept of autonomy, must be the one to facilitate the educational dialogue with the patient in an effort to assist that patient in choosing a treatment plan that aligns with who she is as a separate and distinct individual, even to the detriment of the clinician.

The ideas of therapeutic privilege and waiver have been used to justify the omission of information by the clinician to a patient. Therapeutic privilege is a decision of the clinician to withhold information, whereas waiver is the decision of the patient permitting the clinician to withhold certain types of information. Therapeutic

---

18 President's Commission for the Study of Ethical Problems in Medicine and Biomedical and Behavioral Research. Making Health Care Decisions: The Ethical and Legal Implications of Informed Consent in the Patient- Practitioner Relationship. Vol. 1. Washington: GPO; 1982:39.

19 Ibid., 96.

privilege is often justified by physicians who use it saying that they are protecting their patient from additional or undue stress. However, the President's Commission for the Study of Ethical Problems in Medicine states, "Not only is there no evidence of significant negative psychological consequences of receiving information, but on the contrary some strong evidence indicates that disclosure is beneficial."[20]

Additionally, the definition of waiver is not that the patient suspends or waives the right to informed consent. In fact, if a waiver has actually been obtained, it serves to reinforce informed consent but changes its focus from making decisions about specific treatments with full disclosure to making decisions about what treatment information the patient does not want. "Yet it is questionable whether patients should be permitted to waive the professional's obligation to disclose fundamental information about the nature and implications of certain procedures (such as 'When you wake up, you will learn that your limb has been amputated' or 'You are irreversibly sterile')."[21] To ensure that a waiver has been properly obtained given the questionable nature of its value in light of the potential risk to a patient's self-determination, it would be wise for a physician

---

20 Ibid., 100.

21 Ibid., 94.

to engage a meta-level of informed consent regarding the nature of waiver complete with a signed document verifying that the communication between the clinician and the patient did occur (see Appendix II.B.7: Waiver of Patient Right to Informed Consent).

The use of waiver, even with such clear documentation, contains inherent ethical complexities. Since waiver in its purest form is designed to uphold patient autonomy and self-determination on a meta-level, the use of waiver must be initiated by the patient. For a medical clinician to initiate a waiver suggests a motivation to withhold information or choose a treatment course different from that which the patient is likely to choose.

While the physician may believe he or she acts in the best interest of the patient in initiating waiver, this represents a severe violation of patient autonomy and a conflict of interest for the clinician. However, patients are not likely to know or understand the concept of waiver. Thus, the clinician must rely on cues from the patient which suggest that a waiver could be the desire of the patient, such as: "I don't want to know" "I can't make this decision" "Do whatever you think is best" etc.

Pertinent Standards

(a) Patient Acquisition
Policy stating that the clinician reads through all available patient health history before the patient visit.

Explanation: After the clinician retrieves the patient's prior health history from her primary care physician, he/she tries to clarify the consultative relationship with that physician.

(b) Service

Policy stating that the initial patient visit is for consultation purposes only while patient is in no danger of imminent physical harm, with any treatment to be provided during subsequent visits (treatments for epidemics such as STDs are an exception).

Explanation: The patient's condition is diagnosed by the clinician in graded fashion. If her pregnancy test is positive, then an ultrasound scan is performed to confirm fetal viability and gestational age.

Example: Appendix II.B.9: Medical Exam Report

Policy stating that the clinician is responsible for contextualizing the patient's medical health information.

Explanation: Previous health conditions are gathered by the clinician which could impact the current situation and treatment options, especially past abortion history.

The patient's current health status is determined, including any conditions that would impact treatment options or future reproductive health such as STDs.

All possible side effects (however remote) for all treatment options are identified and communicated in the context of future reproductive health goals and family planning.

Examples: Appendices II.B.10: Initial Visit Health Questionnaire, II.B.11: Excerpt from the CompassCare STD Testing and Treatment Process, II.B.8: Abortion Information Brochure

Policy stating that all treatment options consistent with the patient's context are identified and conveyed in a direct consultation with the clinician.

Explanation: Options presentation includes:

Abortion

Natural miscarriage

Pregnancy termination for fetal demise, including a description of varying procedures by gestational age

Pregnancy termination to save the (physical) life of the mother

Pregnancy termination to save the life of the mother and child

Carry to term Parent child and parent the child

Place child for adoption

Example: Appendix II.B.8: Abortion Information Brochure

Policy stating that non-medical personnel do not provide medical information, and anyone under the supervision of the physician provides only information approved by the physician.

Example: Appendix II.B.12: Confirmation of Pregnancy Policy

Policy stating that the patient is required to sign a waiver of informed consent stating they were made aware of the nature of waiver by the clinician when making the decision to forego the right to information regarding her condition and/or treatment options.

Example: Appendix II.B.7: Waiver of Patient Right to Informed Consent

2. Beneficence

In addition to and support of patient autonomy, the principle of beneficence, according to Beauchamp and Childress, "refers to a statement of moral obligation to act for the benefit of others."[22] This requires the clinician to maintain personal integrity in line with the fundamental virtues noted in The Doctor/Society Relationship below.

a) Continuity of Care

Theory

Continuity of care supports the concept of beneficence and means any treatment is recommended or provided within the larger context of the patient's (1) past health history, (2) current socioeconomic circumstances and personal beliefs, and (3) future health goals. Simply put, it means that the patient is considered as a

---

22 Beauchamp, Childress. *Principles of Biomedical Ethics,* 197.

whole person rather than a disease or a consumer of an isolated medical service. As a patient's health represents a continuum, quality healthcare should take that history and future into consideration. Current decisions will impact or alter future health.

The father of modern medical ethics, Thomas Percival, MD, underscored the importance of total patient engagement, saying, "The feelings and emotions of the patients under critical circumstances require to be known and to be attended to no less than the symptoms of their diseases."[23] For example, an extremely obese man faces social pressures which would be considered a "critical circumstance" and therefore must "be attended to no less than the symptoms" of obesity when exploring weight loss options with the clinician, from habit modification to bariatric surgery. The clinician's first commitment is to the patient as a whole person, which speaks to the ethical principle of beneficence.

Continuity of care comes with the idea that patients can manage their own health care only in conjunction with their primary clinician who is best equipped to understand their beliefs, concerns, and circumstances and how different treatment options relate. As we have

---

23 Percival T. Medical Ethics; Or a Code of Institutes and Precepts Adapted to the Professional Conduct of Physicians and Surgeons. Manchester: S. Russell; 1803:10.

seen, understanding patients is essential to helping guide them to the appropriate treatment plan and understand if any specialist should be consulted.

Accepting and treating a patient as a specialist outside of the patient's primary clinician in non-emergent, elective circumstances can violate the basic principle of beneficence. This is true because a specialist simply cannot know the patient's health history, personal beliefs, and circumstances well enough to know that the treatment option provided by that specialist would be the one that is in the best interest of the patient—especially if the treatment option provided by the specialist is the most invasive of all treatment options (see Prevention). As the American College of Physicians notes, "The consultant should respect the relationship between the patient and the principal physician, should promptly and effectively communicate recommendations to the principal physician, and should obtain concurrence of the principle physician for major procedures or additional consultants."[24]

Therefore, a patient's request for specialized medical services should be a cue to that clinician that he may be dealing with an ethical dilemma. For example, no ethical bariatric surgeon would agree to perform gastric bypass simply upon a patient's request with-

---

24 American College of Physicians. *Ethics Manual,* 589.

out contacting the patient's primary care clinician and holding a consultation with the patient to ensure that they have explored all possible causes and exhausted all other less invasive options. It is incumbent upon the specialist to ensure continuity of care by engaging the patient's primary care clinician in situations like these (see Pertinent Standards for detailed policies designed to ensure continuity of care). Not to do so is to ignore the ethical concept of beneficence and could harm the patient by violating her autonomy. Additionally, this mandate to maintain continuity of care provides a measure of clinician accountability for the specialist to avoid the conflict of interest inherent in specialization beyond what any legislative body could ensure.

To further keep the patient from harm by the clinician, accurate documentation of patient care is necessary to ensure two-way communication toward informed consent (Autonomy) and continuity of care (Beneficence). As Southard and Frankel state, "The importance of accurate and comprehensive documentation on every medical record should not be underestimated."[25] Absent access to a patient's record, a clinician cannot foster continuity of care.

---

25 Southard P, Frankel P. Trauma care documentation: A comprehensive guide. *J Emerg Nurs.* 1989;15(5):393.

Pertinent Standards

(a) Patient Acquisition

Policy stating that it is communicated to the patient that the first appointment is to diagnose her condition and explore all treatment options.

Example: Appendices II.B.13: Limitations of Services, II.B.14: What Can You Expect? Form

Policy stating that if the patient was acquired through a referral from her primary care physician, the clinician attempts to attain her health record and/or a brief discussion with that physician regarding the patient's background and the reason for the referral.

Example: Appendices B: Tools for Ethical Decision-making in the Context of Reproductive Health Services, II.B.15: Authorization for Release of Medical Information

(b) Service

Policy stating that if the patient was acquired through advertising with no referral from her primary care physician, the clinician is to engage the patient with a health history questionnaire and situational assessment.

Explanation: The clinician attempts to clarify with the patient the role of her primary care physician.

Example: Appendices II.B.4: Patient Intake Form, II.B.10: Initial Visit Health Questionnaire

(c) Follow-up

Policy stating that all patients will be referred back to their primary care physician after specialist consultation to pursue treatment options.

Explanation: Patient will be given "Next Steps" and referrals information including a scheduled follow-up appointment when indicated.

Example: Appendix II.B.5: Personalized Solutions Assessment

Policy stating that all treatment options include appropriate post-treatment follow-up

Explanation:

Surgical treatments immediate observation

Post-surgical emergency access

General, post-surgery in-office follow-up

Medicinal treatments

At least the follow-up described in the recommendations of the FDA, the drug company, or state department of health, whichever is most stringent.

Natural Treatments

The clinician ensures that the patient acquires appropriate prenatal care.

Examples: Appendices II.B.16: FDA Mifeprex Medication Guide, II.B.17: Sample Follow-up Process

Policy stating that the closing procedure for patient records is followed in every case

Example: Appendix II.B.18: Closing Summary Form

Accurate Documentation

Policy stating that all patient care will be documented in full and will include the patient's primary care clinician, values, circumstances and contraindicated options, the delivery of community-support referrals, and a follow-up plan.

Examples: Appendix II.B.5: Personalized Solutions Assessment

The types of files which may be included in a comprehensive patient chart are listed in Appendix.II.B.19: Patient Chart Outline.

b) No Conflict of Interest

Theory

Maintaining no conflict of interest involves the protection of the patient from any intentional or unintentional clinician self-interest (anything that places the clinician's needs or desires above the patient's), including finances, beliefs about the nature of humanity, etc. Only the clinician can ensure this. It requires critical self-reflection by clinicians to accurately identify their own interests.

Thinking first of the patient in all matters is reinforced by the notion of no conflict of interest. Financial conflict of interest is certainly one aspect of the issue whereby a clinician would be placed in a circumstance of acting in ways counter to the best interests of the patient. This fact remains supported today: "Although the physician should be fairly compensated for services rendered, a sense of duty to the patient should take precedence over concern about compensation when a patient's well-being is at stake."[26]

During the course of the development of modern medicine and the complexities it represents, the profession has seen fit to foster an educational environment whereby a clinician can specialize in caring for a particular part of the human anatomy and even further specialize in treatments or procedures unique to that specialty.

Typically, these types of treatments or procedures require clinicians dedicated to performing only those procedures either because of their complexity or the high demand for that service. This specialization produces some valuable efficiency when distributing limited medical resources to the general public (see Distributive Justice) but also carries with it potential for conflict of interest if the patient chooses a course of treatment that does not include the specific services offered by that specialist. In the example of the obese man, the bariatric surgeon and the dietician both have vested interest in a particular treatment option which must be communicated before his choice of treatment. Also, if the services of the specialist represent a fundamental

---

26 American College of Physicians. *Ethics Manual,* 577.

difference in a patient's transcendent beliefs, a conflict of interest would also be present. So if this obese man was a Christian Scientist who believed it wrong to engage any direct medicinal or surgical intervention, the only proper action toward a solution would be an identification of the conflicts of interest in a candid process of communication and an exploration of those potential conflicts by the specialist himself with the patient.

Pertinent Standards

(a) Patient Acquisition

Policy stating that the clinician will not schedule a treatment or procedure without a prior medical consultation.

Explanation: Due to the emotional context of abortion, the clinician treats each patient as an ethical dilemma and asks the question of him- or herself, "Should we provide an abortion to this patient?" Every initial patient visit will help the patient explore all of her treatment options.

(b) Service

Policy stating that the clinician must communicate verbally and in writing his/her potential bias toward any treatment option.

Explanation: The clinician discloses any financial interest in a particular treatment option.

Example: See statement of financial interest in Appendix II.B.13: Limitations of Services

Policy declaring the clinician's values, which may differ from those of the patient.

Explanation: Clinician identifies personal values pertaining to all issues related to pregnancy options including his/her belief as to when human life begins.

Example: See statement of values regarding abortion in Appendix II.B.13: Limitations of Services

(c) Follow-up

Policy stating that a standard follow-up process is used for every patient.

Explanation: The patient is treated with equal respect regardless of the treatment option chosen.

3. Non-maleficence

Non-maleficence is the physician's attempt to avoid any act or treatment plan that would harm the patient or violate the patient's trust. Non-maleficence and beneficence in many respects represent two sides of the same coin. If beneficence means to act in the best interest of the patient, then non-maleficence ensures that the patient is not harmed in any way by the relationship and activities of the doctor. This ethical idea is often stated as "First, do no harm." In a clinician's zeal to heal, he may overlook certain aspects of the patient's condition and inadvertently hurt that patient either in the short or long run. The concept of non-maleficence ideally encourages a doctor to think in a more circumspect manner about who the patient is and what her circumstances are, as well as understanding and respecting her wishes, before rushing too quickly to judgment and treatment.

For example, if a patient believes that a fetus represents a separate and distinct human being, then it is incumbent upon the clinician, irrespective of his beliefs, to recognize and respect the autonomy of a second patient, the child, through the surrogacy of the mother. The Hippocratic Oath as translated by Kass says it this way: "I will keep [patients] from harm and injustice."[27] To refuse to recognize the beliefs about humanity held by the patient as bona fide and relevant to the decision-making process is to place the clinician above the patient. If the patient is uncertain about what she believes, it is critical that the clinician not make any assumptions. Based on the concept of non-maleficence, in this case the clinician must facilitate a candid conversation about fetal development and the nature of pregnancy termination—the separation of the child from the mother for the purpose of fetal demise.

a) Prevention

Theory

---

27 Hippocrates. *The Hippocratic Oath.* Trans. in Kass LR. *Toward a More Natural Science.* New York: Simon and Schuster; 1988:228-9.

Prevention means helping the patient maintain good health to avoid deteriorating conditions and ensuring that all less invasive treatment options are considered before recommending higher-risk measures. "The need of the physician is twofold: preserving health and curing disease, and the demand for the former is greater than for the latter, for it is better for man that he avoid becoming ill than that he become ill and be cured."[28]

The first aspect of prevention includes communicating to the patient about positive lifestyle practices as well as recommending preventative treatments such as vaccinations. The ethical principle of prevention also requires the clinician to encourage the exploration of all less invasive and therefore less risky treatment options available for the patient's condition. Returning to the example of the obese man, the bariatric surgeon is ethically constrained to ensure that the patient has considered all less risky treatments before performing gastric bypass surgery (see Pertinent Standards for further practical policies and examples of upholding non-maleficence through prevention).

If a clinician is not working first toward prevention, he cannot be seen as upholding the ethical concept of non-maleficence. As an example, in the field of re-

---

28 Friedenwald H. The ethics of the practice of medicine from the Jewish point of view. Bulletin of the John Hopkins Hospital. 1917;28(318):258.

productive health when a patient chooses to have an abortion, the clinician should ensure that appropriate sexually transmitted disease testing and treatment has been performed to lower the risk of infection and future reproductive health complications.[29]

Pertinent Standards

(a) Patient Acquisition

Policy stating that the clinician never assumes that the patient understands treatment options and always assists the patient in exploring less invasive treatment options first.

(b) Service

Policy stating that least invasive options are encouraged first.

Explanation: For a patient with a negative pregnancy test, offer a discussion around lifestyle measures that

---

29 Ovigstad E, Skaug K, Jerve F, Fylling P, Ulstrup JC. Pelvic inflammatory disease associated with Chlamydia trachomatis infection after therapeutic abortion: A prospective study. *Br J Vener Dis.* 1983;59(3):189-92; Westergaard L, Philipsen T, Scheibel J. Significance of cervical Chlamydia trachomatis infection in postabortal pelvic inflammatory disease. *Obstet Gynecol.* 1982;60(3):322-5; Chacko MR, Lovchik JC. Chiamydia trachomatis infection in sexually active adolescents: Prevalence and risk factors. *Pediatrics.* 1984;73(6):836-40; Barbacci MB, Spence M, Kappus EW, Murkman RC, Rao L, Quinn TC. Postabortal endometritis and isolation of Chlamydia trachomatis. *Obstet Gynecol.* 1986;68(5):686-90; Duthie SJ, Hobson D, Tait IA, Pratt BC, Lowe N, Sequeira PJ, et al. Morbidity after termination of pregnancy in first trimester. *Genitourin Med.* 1987;63(3):182-7.

reduce risk of unplanned pregnancy and STDs. For a patient with a positive pregnancy test, offer a discussion around abortion and additional health implications post-abortion, adoption, parenting, the nature of birth control, and related education for healthy lifestyle measures.

Examples: Appendices II.B.20: STD Education Script, II.B.21: STD Education Worksheet

Information to support prevention education is included in Appendix II.B.22: Health Questionnaire Breakdown.

Policy stating that all STD testing and treatment will occur before any treatment options are provided relative to pregnancy to protect mother's future reproductive health and her child.

b) Confidentiality

Theory

Finally, the idea of confidentiality is critical in safe-guarding a patient from harm and injustice. Confidentiality is simply maintaining the privacy of all patient information. This is important to the clinician/ patient relationship because it is the construct which allows the free and complete flow of communication from the patient to the doctor. Only then can the doctor educate the patient toward prevention and appropriate treatment plans. If the patient does not believe confidentiality will be maintained, then he/she will withhold key pieces of information necessary for a complete and accurate diagnosis and options presentation.

Since we as a society believe in the autonomy and therefore the dignity of the individual, it remains that all aspects of patient care be kept in the strictest confidence. In the United States, the Federal Government expresses this value through its 1996 Health Insurance Portability and Accountability Act (HIPAA), which attempts to guarantee that the minimum amount of patient data needed for patient care is transmitted between parties and only at the permission of the patient. While HIPAA regulations are complex and compliance itself has become an industry, policies evolving directly from the basic ethical principle of non-maleficence as described in Pertinent Standards below ensure compliance with traditional medical ethics.

Pertinent Standards

(a) Patient Acquisition

Policy stating that all clinician staff will maintain total confidentiality of patient records except where prohibited by law.

Explanation: The patient is told that all records will be held confidential.

Example: The confidentiality statement in Appendix II.B.6: Patient Bill of Rights

(b) Service

Policy stating that all patients are asked to sign a release of records for the clinician to engage her primary care physician or a third-party payer.

Example: Appendices II.B.23: Confidentiality Policy and Procedure, II.B.15: Authorization for Release of Medical Information

(c) Follow-up

Policy stating that diagnostic results will be delivered in person, to the extent possible; all electronic transfer of patient information must be safeguarded through encryption or other means.

B. The Doctor/Society Relationship

As medicine has been practiced for centuries throughout the world, it represents an almost universally respected discipline. The name for the discipline's primary practitioner is "doctor" which emanates from the Latin root "to teach:" *docere*. The implications of this nomenclature are important with respect to the role of the clinician within society as foremost patient advocate.

Because society has given such an implicit trust to the role of clinician, the profession has endeavored to protect that trust through the generations by identifying and being held accountable to standards of ethical conduct professionally as well as personally. In fact, one of the earliest and perhaps most widely known professional commitments of care is the Hippocratic Oath.

Through the years the Oath has been modified and used to varying degrees in the education of medical professionals. Based on the ancient Hippocratic Oath, "Medical Ethics" was developed, a phrase originally attributed to an English physician, Thomas Percival, who wrote *Medical Ethics: or a Code of the Institutes and Precepts Adapted to the Professional Conduct of Physicians and Surgeons,* first published in 1794. This code was later used as the basis for the American Medical Association's Code of Ethics in 1846.

As religious belief, science, medicine, law, and government have become more involved in the management and delivery of medicine, the notion of Medical Ethics has grown into a more comprehensive discipline now known as bioethics. This relatively new field attempts to identify—and in some cases solve—the ethical dilemmas that occur where medical practice interfaces with society's new technologies, changing cultural mores, government regulation, etc.

So for a clinician to hold preeminent the patient, he must consider his relationship with society, and society in turn must consider its relationship to the medical community. Society has entrusted the medical community with the most basic physical manifestation of itself: a solitary life. Medicine represents an unstated contract with society, whereby society entrusts the lives of her people to the clinician, and the clinician in turn carries a duty to objectively care without respect to social or financial status, a concept known as distributive justice. Therefore, questions of the nature of humanity and the definition of its limits are interwoven in issues of economics, legislation, education, research, and technology.

In the midst of the sea of complexity float issues of reproductive health. Issues of human reproduction resurface time and again in virtually every setting where medicine touches research, government, religion, and even economics. This is the case, certainly in part if not in whole, due to the fact that it represents the very foundation and definition of that for which medicine exists: the health of a single human. It is because of this fundamental reality that reproductive health issues and services must be handled without presumption or transference of belief on a case-by-case basis with utmost delicacy.

Because the practice of medicine happens within a changing culture and is performed by men and women who are a product of that culture, it is paramount that physicians and other medical practitioners understand and teach society how the practice of medicine can and must occur in the context of differing personal or political beliefs. This is done by understanding the concepts that govern the relationship a doctor has with society. Those concepts have traditionally been personal integrity, distributive justice, and education.

1. Clinician Personal Integrity

A clinician's personal commitment to integrity is essential to the medical community to maintain its credibility with the society it serves. Without it, trust and honesty cannot be maintained, destroying the most basic bond a society has with medicine: the doctor/patient relationship. Absent this bond the clinician is unable to consistently and accurately collect and interpret the information needed from the patient to effectively educate toward prevention or treatment options consistent with the patient's values. The clinician's personal commitment to integrity has always been part and parcel to his relationship to society as stated in the original Hippocratic Oath: "In purity and holiness I will guard my life and my art."[30] In fact, maintaining personal integrity is so closely linked with maintaining medicine's contract with society that even the mere perception of impropriety should be avoided: "Trust in the profession is undermined when there is even the appearance of impropriety."[31]

a) Virtue

Patients cannot be expected to know and understand the basic ethical criteria of medical decision-

---

30 Hippocrates. *The Hippocratic Oath.* Trans. in Kass.

31 American College of Physicians. *Ethics Manual,* 587.

making; governments cannot be expected to have the scope of power and expertise required to protect its citizens from malpractice. As a result, the clinician has been endowed tremendous power. Since a patient can be easily manipulated due to their lack of knowledge, it requires that the clinician be personally virtuous, committed to wisdom, empathy, temperance, courage, and justice. Absent a clinician's personal dedication to virtue, patients are doomed to a fate of exploitation and victimization for the personal gain of the clinician (perhaps without even the clinician's awareness). This lack of virtue represents a moral bankruptcy actively abusing the implicit contract and sacred trust a society has with its medical community.

Basic medical-ethical decision-making can only be driven by the clinician. So to disregard or even downplay the personal character of the clinician in the clinician/patient relationship would be tantamount to driving a car without a steering wheel. The following is a list of classical virtues born out of early Greek philosophy and in many ways reinforced by the Judeo-Christian belief system within which Western medicine was fostered:

i. Wisdom (and Shrewd Stewardship): The passion to seek knowledge for the purpose of effectively managing resources to solve problems.

ii. Empathy (and Social Intelligence): The commitment to understanding the emotions a person experiences in association with certain life situations in an effort to engage that situation with intelligence and compassion.

iii. Temperance (and Self-Regulation): The ability to regulate feelings and actions in order to put another's needs ahead of one's own desires.

iv. Courage (and Honesty): The willingness to self-reflect and the ability to take responsibility or to genuinely own up to one's own attitudes, behaviors, and limitations.

v. Justice (and Leadership): The commitment to the ordering of people and other resources with accountability on behalf of those unable to do so for themselves.

The underlying concept to all of the above virtues is self-sacrifice for the benefit and well-being of others. Only when clinicians are committed to this degree of personal virtue can the traditional concepts of ethical decision-making in the clinician/patient relationship be consistently and meaningfully invoked.

b) Clinician Right of Conscience

Clinician conscience rights in the arena of reproductive health services have been a topic of healthy debate in recent years. In fact, the American College of Obstetricians and Gynecologists issued Committee Opinion 385 in 2007 defining what they described as "appropriate limits of conscientious refusal"[32] of treatment. This overemphasizes patient autonomy, inappropriately creating a right to demand services at least equal to the patient's right to refuse treatment. A patient's right to demand a service as rationale to override a physician's right to refuse treatment relegates medicine to a consumer service and largely ignores a physician's duty to be ethically circumspect on behalf of the patient to consider treatment options with the patient using the ethical notions beneficence and non-maleficence. An excellent Critique of ACOG Committee Opinion #385 by Dr. Robert Orr can be found at www.consciencelaws.org/issues-ethical/ethical079b.htm.

It is within the notion of a clinician's commitment to personal integrity that a society must support and applaud the ethical notion of a Clinician's Right of Conscience to refuse treatment. Without the ability of the clinician to refuse to perform medicine that compromises his personal integrity, society itself would be damaging the foundation of the trust it keeps in the medical community. This fact has been buttressed by the President's Commission on Making Health Care Decisions: "Similarly, a professional who has been as flexible about possible avenues of treatment as his or

---

32 American College of Obstetricians and Gynecologists. The limits of conscientious refusal in reproductive medicine. ACOG Committee Opinion No. 385. *Obstet Gynecol.* 2007;110(5):1204.

her beliefs and standards allow is not generally obligated to accede to the patient in a way that violates the bounds of acceptable medical practice or the provider's own deeply held moral beliefs."[33] In an article published recently in the *British Medical Journal* relating to the reasonable physician standard for conscientious refusal of abortion services in the US, most OB/GYNs supported the physician's right of conscientious refusal stating in the conclusion that "the majority of OB/GYNS support physicians conscientiously refusing to perform an abortion . . ."[34]

2. Distributive Justice

Another key ethical category that has served to govern the doctor/society relationship is distributive justice. This concept recognizes the limited resources of the medical community; there are always more patient needs to serve than medicine can accommodate. Therefore, the American College of Physicians holds that the concept "requires that we seek to equitably distribute the life-enhancing opportunities afforded by

---

33 President's Commission. Making health care decisions, 38.

34 Rasinski KA, Yoon JD, Kalad YG, Curlin FA. Obstetrician- gynaecologists' opinions about conscientious refusal of a request for abortion: results from a national vignette experiment. *J Med Ethics.* Published online 13 Jun 2011 [cited 2 Nov 2011]. Available from: http://jme.bmj.com/content/early/2011/06/13/jme.2010.040782.abstract?sid=306877bb-775d-4c9b-bdcc-30acbab50b92

health care."[35] Unfortunately, there has been clash in recent years over access to elective reproductive health services like abortion as an issue of appropriate medical resource allocation. Abortion proponents argue that a clinician electing a right to refuse treatment impedes access to needed or standard reproductive health medicine, the assumption being that issues of conscience are merely personal opinion and should be set aside when a patient either does not have the resources or the reasonable geographic proximity to a physician that will provide one. This position presumes that the moral opinion of those holding to the notion that abortion actually represents ethical medicine should be the default moral position of all physicians in certain circumstances.

Because of the immediate nature of medical care, it is neither political lobbying groups, legislative or governing bodies, nor any other group in society that is equipped to distribute medical resources. Rather, it is the medical community alone that is able to understand the needs of the society at large and understand the best means to equitably distribute those resources for her care without violating medical ethics. The sweeping hand of government is unable to do so due to its lack of medical training in the understanding of medical service delivery. It can only support medicine at its best.

---

35 American College of Physicians. *Ethics Manual*, 577.

Medicine has been the topic and target of reform in recent years in the United States. These reforms generally emanate from state or federal government and of late have focused primarily on issues of adequate distribution of medical services. The difficulty that inevitably arises when medicine is legislated by those outside the practice of it is an imbalanced focus or overemphasis on one particular aspect of medical service over others. Making distributive justice of primary importance to a physician, for example, can hinder that physician from his first duty to focus on his patient's needs. This inadvertently makes the legislative body or the prevailing political agenda the primary relationship to the physician rather than the patient. Only an ethical physician and the medical community can determine how best to distribute the resources of medicine appropriately.

Government may need to intervene to protect its citizens from the abuse of clinicians whose personal integrity is compromised. It is here that the government must take care to keep from being manipulated by morally defective, self-interested clinicians. Such may attempt to create legislation for their own benefit, which would force medicine outside the bounds of traditional ethical practice and create scenarios that reinforce unethical discriminatory practices or the restriction of the availability of needed ethical medical services.

3. Education: Propagation of the Art and Informing Society

A final key ethical category managing the doctor/society relationship is education, both to inform society at large as to how medicine should be applied and also to teach the next generation of clinicians the art of medicine. One modern version of the Hippocratic Oath puts it this way: "I will respect the hard-won scientific gains of those physicians in whose steps I walk, and gladly share such knowledge as is mine with those who are to follow."[36]

The American College of Physicians goes on to say, "Society looks to physicians to establish professional standards of practice."[37] A clinician has an obligation not just to help educate the next generation of clinicians about the nature and practice of medicine but he also has a responsibility to protect society's most vulnerable. This is done not only through the practice of distributive justice but also by educating legislatures and litigators as expert witnesses, acting as guardians of the disenfranchised against self-interested others even if that means testifying against other clinicians.

This level of professional accountability requires the maintenance of high personal integrity because the

36 Lasagna L. A Modern Hippocratic Oath. 1964 [cited 3 Aug 2011]. Available from: http://www.aapsonline.org/ethics/oaths.htm#lasagna

37 American College of Physicians. *Ethics Manual*, 590.

practice of medicine and its interaction with society is facilitated by the doctor. This is the case primarily because society at large lacks the education and expertise to engage issues of medical service in as comprehensive and circumspect a manner as clinicians themselves. So when society needs to engage through legislation or litigation an issue that concerns medicine, it is a clinician's ethical obligation to treat that engagement as an expert witness with the same level of gravity that he would bring to an individual patient. Louise Andrew aptly states:

> Because most expert medical witness testimony about the performance of physicians requires that a witness be medically licensed, and because verdicts based on expert testimony directly influence the standard of care that will be applied in the future, providing medical testimony legitimately can be considered to come within the realm of the practice of medicine. Testifying as an expert in legal matters should be undertaken with the same degree of integrity as the practice of medicine and is rightfully subject to the same degree of scrutiny and regulation.[38]

It is toward responsibility to the society at large for a physician and the body of clinicians in the medical

---

38 Andrew LB. Expert witness testimony: The ethics of being a medical expert witness. *Emerg Med Clin North Am.* 2006; 24(3):715.

community that this document and the following tools are offered. Too often polls are conducted asking the general population about their feelings on the nature of abortion when in fact the wrong questions are being asked. The right questions can only be asked in the context of a meaningful clinician/patient relationship. Furthermore, the answers to the right questions should not be legislated unless they obviously concern a categorical and consistent violation of the ubiquitous respect for the life, liberty, and security of the citizenry.

II. Standards of Practice

Medical Care Process Chain

The practice of medicine in a clinician/patient relationship largely represents an iterative process including data collection (patient to doctor and doctor to patient), data analysis, diagnosis, education on treatment options, and determination of a treatment plan. Often, once an initial round of data collection and analysis has taken place, it becomes clear that more data must be collected and analyzed in order to appropriately educate patients, diagnose their conditions, and recommend treatment plans consistent with their beliefs and values.

Data collection includes the clinician collecting data from the patient. This represents not only information related the patient's immediate presentation symptoms but also information about the patient's behavior, beliefs, and personal circumstances—social and otherwise—that would impact a patient's treatment plan. If the clinician is a specialist, then part of data collection would include securing the assent of the patient's primary clinician to act as her consultant in caring for her patient. This relationship can then be used to insure that the patient's decision about treatment options remains free and uncoerced by either the clinician or her circumstances. Data collection also occurs by the patient in the education of her condition by the clinician and how her goals, circumstances, and values might relate to the available treatment options.

After data has been collected, it must be reviewed or analyzed in conjunction with the patient. This not only educates the clinician about the specific case of the patient but also serves to educate the patient so as to be able to make a treatment choice that is truly informed. Once the clinician believes he has sufficient information to make a diagnosis, he does so by communicating that diagnosis to the patient and by officially documenting it in the patient's record.

When the patient's condition is finally diagnosed, treatment options are communicated. It is here that the clinician must leverage the data he has collected about the patient's beliefs and personal circumstances in an effort to avoid a transcendent, financial, or any other conflict of interest. This means the clinician must know what he believes to such a degree as not to influence the patient to make a decision that is inconsistent with what she believes. Also, if a patient's circumstances represent possible emotional distress and coercion through relationships pushing her toward a treatment option that is inconsistent with her beliefs, it is the doctor's responsibility to insulate her from those things through active communication.

Finally, a treatment plan should be decided upon by the patient. At that time a determination is made as to whether the clinician will be involved in that plan. The clinician should be confident that the patient has made a choice that is consistent with her beliefs, free from coercion, and in the context of her primary clinician relationship. Additionally, if the patient has made a treatment choice that violates the clinician's own deeply held convictions, her conscience would dictate—and society must support—her right to refuse treatment.

Legislation or policy placing an expectation upon a clinician to violate her conscience undermines the clinician's integrity and ability to uphold the basic ethical categories that govern the clinician/patient relationship.

In the realm of reproductive health, specialty clinicians of pregnancy services must be aware that most of their patients request services without consulting their primary clinician and are in emotional distress. It is of paramount importance that such clinicians understand the standing medical-ethical dilemma that each separate patient represents and work diligently to ensure that the treatment plan upholds and is consistent with the three basic ethical categories for direct patient care. For a specialty clinician to assume that any of the above steps have taken place without consulting the patient's primary clinician—or at least actively engaging in a healthy give-and-take conversation with the patient—could harm the patient by subverting her true autonomy.

It bears restating that "Society looks to physicians to establish professional standards of practice."[39] This is so because it is only they who can apply their knowledge and expertise to a patient without violating the basic trust they have with society and with their patients. It is precisely their understanding of medicine and how it should be practiced that makes them only and uniquely suited to determine the standard for patient care both at the societal and individual level. It is the body of clinicians that can hold themselves accountable to these standards because they alone can determine and verify sub-par or unethical performance in a colleague as expert witnesses, etc.

Standards of practice represent how a patient should be treated in certain circumstances taking into consideration all elements of medical ethics for service delivery: autonomy, beneficence, and non-maleficence. To reflect upon and hold to ethical standards of care requires the personal integrity of the clinician and the proper education of that clinician by the generation of clinicians that preceded him. Without this personal commitment to virtue, it is unlikely a clinician could

39 American College of Physicians. *Ethics Manual*, 590.

consistently apply the medical ethics necessary that represent respectful, ethical patient care.

It has been the observation of this commission that practice of traditional and ethical medicine has been compromised in the medical specialty of Reproductive Health Services through self-interested organizations, specialty clinicians, and ill-informed legislators. Our times of polarized and sensationalized political battle within this important field of medicine require a set of objective ethical standards with historical and apolitical foundations—standards which ensure that each patient is treated with the dignity she deserves by protecting her self-determination, standards which ensure clinicians are once more venerated in their noble place as servant-healers rather than technicians providing a consumer product.

Appendices

A. Controlling Beliefs and the Idea of Transcendent Authority

The belief of the intrinsic value of humanity has traditionally been rooted in a transcendent authority "that they are endowed by their Creator with certain unalienable Rights, that among these are Life, Liberty, and the pursuit of Happiness."[40] This transcendent belief is the basis for principles of the nature and beliefs about the essence of humanity. These beliefs inform ethical concepts driving moral behavior—how individuals should act within society. The concept of transcendence represents what Aristotle termed "first causes"[41] or, in other words, an absolute authority. Given that fact, it must be noted that all absolute authority is circular as to the rationale for its validity, since by definition absolute authority cannot be conferred lest it be subservient to the authority that conferred it.

---

40 Declaration of Independence.

41 Aristotle. *Metaphysics*. Trans. Ross. 1.1.7

Even in the original Hippocratic Oath, the gods are invoked as authoritative witnesses overseeing the blessing of those who keep the oath and the punishment for those that fail to uphold it, stating, "I swear by Apollo the physician, and Asclepius, and Hygieia and Panacea and all the gods and goddesses as my witnesses, that, according to my ability and judgment, I will keep this Oath and this contract."[42] Understanding transcendence in medicine is essential to keeping the clinician from "play[ing] at God"[43] or becoming her own transcendent authority, thereby compromising the primary protection of the patient's autonomy. Therefore, the idea of transcendence for the clinician to maintain objectivity and consistency is critical in order to keep from doing harm (non-maleficence) and to uphold the patient as preeminent (beneficence) in the acts of understanding, diagnosing, educating, and treating. It has been said that all decisions are moral ones since each one presupposes a belief complete with a stated or unstated final authority, be it the Greek pantheon, the Judeo-Christian Jehovah, or the Kantian enlightenment notion of human reason and observation sufficient for all human enquiry.

---

42 Hippocrates. *The Hippocratic Oath*. Trans. North M. National Library of Medicine; 2002 [cited 3 Nov 2011]. Available from: http://www.nlm.nih.gov/hmd/greek/greek_oath.html

43 Lasagna. A Modern Hippocratic Oath.

It is the transcendent belief of the intrinsic value of a single human being that informs the clinician/patient relationship through the ethical principles of autonomy, beneficence, and non-maleficence. A commitment to hold preeminent the patient through these principles remains incumbent upon each clinician. This idea of patient preeminence is traditionally articulated through an intentional and objective process of understanding and supporting the patient by fostering communication and treatment plans consistent with the patient's belief system, insulating them from those of the clinician should they differ. This is especially true when it comes to the beliefs about the nature of human life both as it pertains to its end and its beginning. Though thoughts and beliefs about the ultimate reason for human existence are personal, they impact the decisions we make about how we interact with the people and world around us. Because clinicians are products of the society they presume to serve, they must be self-aware to such an extent so as not to inappropriately leverage their knowledge and position influencing a patient to their own personal belief, agenda, or financial gain.

B. Tools for Ethical Decision-Making in the Context of Reproductive Health Services

The following tools are designed to assist the medical community insulating women and their children from the exploitation of self-interested political voices and clinicians willing to provide medical services outside of traditional and current medical-ethical standards.

1. Ethical Dilemma Indicators

In an effort to assist the medical community, the judicial system, and legislative bodies, the following list of indicators revealing potential ethical clinical dilemmas is provided. These are only indicators that would cue a clinician to the possibility that a patient presentation may represent an ethical dilemma according to existing standards of medical ethics and practice. They are not intended to be exhaustive but instead assist the clinician toward a more ethical engagement of a patient in a society divided on this issue of abortion often apart from informed ethical medicine.

Autonomy

1. Patient is unwilling to engage a discussion about various treatment options—she has apparently already made up her mind without clinician dialogue (Informed Consent).

2. Patient is unwilling to communicate about her beliefs regarding the nature of a human or fetal development (Informed Consent).

3. Patient is emotionally distressed, which could imply relational coercion (Self-Determination).

4. Patient is not interested in understanding the extent of her condition (Informed Consent).

Beneficence

1. Patient requests a specific medical procedure without clinician consultation (Continuity of Care).

2. Patient presents to clinician without primary clinician referral (Continuity of Care).

3. Patient has not consulted with her primary clinician (Continuity of Care).

4. Clinician is tempted not to engage the patient in a circumspect and candid conversation because of a possible difference in transcendent belief if it meant he would not be able to provide a treatment option (Conflict of Interest).

Non-maleficence

1. Patient is unwilling to participate in or impatient with the medical care process (Prevention).

2. Patient expresses heightened concern about confidentiality extending even to health insurance and primary care clinician knowledge (Confidentiality).

3. Patient believes that a pregnancy represents a human life obligating the clinician to recognize surrogacy and opts for an abortion anyway (Prevention/Clinician Personal Integrity).

2. Clinical-Ethical Decision-Making Steps

Based on the nature of abortion services and the manner in which a patient typically accesses them, it seems that the very environment of reproductive health services creates an ethical dilemma on a per patient basis. This being the case, it is helpful to note how other medical clinicians deal with ethical decision-making. The American College of Physicians has provided a helpful eight-step process "To Assist Clinical Ethics Decision-Making."[44] The steps are as follows (direct quotes in italics):

1. Define the ethics problem as an "ought" or "should" question.

Example: Should we provide an abortion to this patient?

NOT: Should abortion be legal? Or Is this pregnant woman an ethics problem?

2. List significant facts and uncertainties that are relevant to the question. Include facts about the patient and care givers (such as intimacy, emotional state, ethnic and cultural background, and faith traditions)

Example: This woman has been living with her boyfriend for five months and is a Catholic. She is emotion-

---

44 American College of Physicians. *Ethics Manual*, 592-3.

ally unstable because she is afraid her boyfriend would not be supportive and that her parents will stop paying for her college education should she have the baby.

3. Identify a decision-maker.

Example: Patient is competent, of age, and has not been deemed mentally unstable by a court or has been emancipated either by legal category or by specific court decision and therefore is the decision-maker for her own health.

4. Give understandable, relevant, desired information to the decision-maker and dispel myths and misconceptions.

Example: A pregnancy always ends with the separation of the child from the mother, usually by natural means through miscarriage or natural birth. Other times a pregnancy ends through direct medical intervention for either one of three reasons: (1) To save the lives of both mother and child, (2) to save the life of the mother, or (3) to end the life of the child, generally referred to as "abortion." A child in the womb has distinctly different DNA from the mother which controls and determines its own development starting at conception all the way through until mature human death. The gestational age of a child typically determines characteristics of fetal development and would therefore impact the type of abortion procedure the patient would be eligible to receive. Some abortion procedures are illegal, and all carry with them risks and side effects. Examples of side effects through peer-reviewed medical journals would be an increased relative risk of future pre-term deliveries[45] and an increased relative risk of breast cancer.[46]

5. Solicit values of the patient that are relevant to the question.

Example: What are your values about life, such as when do you believe it begins? If the patient believes or has a cultural/faith tradition that holds to human life beginning at conception, it is morally imperative that the clinician explore that. If the patient is uncertain, the clinician is obligated to educate in such a way so as not to sway the patient toward a view inconsistent with their beliefs or toward a view that would financially benefit the clinician.

NOT: Do you think you should have an abortion?

6. Identify health professional values. Values include those related to both the doctor/society relationship and the doctor/patient relationship.

---

45 Rooney B, Calhoun BC. Induced abortion and risk of later premature births. *J Am Phys Surg.* 2003;8(2):46-9.

46 Daling JR, Malone KE, Voigt LF, White E, Weiss NS. Risk of breast cancer among young women: Relationship to induced abortion. *J Natl Cancer Inst.* 1994;86(21):1584-92.

Example: Although the clinician may believe that abortion is indicated for this woman presenting with unplanned pregnancy, the patient has voiced a faith background and emotionally coercive circumstances that would compromise her autonomy; therefore, the clinician cannot in good conscience perform the procedure.

NOT: The patient has signed a legal document stating she understands her options and the risks involved in the procedure chosen.

7. Propose and critique solutions, including multiple options for treatment and alternative clinicians.

Example: The physician, in protecting the interests and values of this patient who cannot speak on his own behalf (the pregnant woman's developing baby by virtue of the mother's transcendent beliefs), must serve as the patient's advocate to the parents of the patient. Therefore, treatment options for pre-natal care and patient transfer/referral must be arranged.

NOT: Clinician will do whatever patient decides.

8. Identify and remove or address constraints on solutions (such as reimbursement, unavailability of services, laws, or legal myths).

Example: The patient cannot afford pre-natal care and cannot continue her education if she has a baby. The clinician notes a full state medical-aid program for pregnant mothers in her age group and is able to connect her with a social worker who will help connect her with child care support for college students.

3. Bill of Rights for Women Facing Unintended Pregnancy

A Woman Facing Unintended Pregnancy Has The Right To:

1. Receive services in a non-judgmental, caring environment committed to maintaining confidentiality of patient records except where required by law.

2. Receive professional medical services from organizations and medical professionals committed to integrity, free from manipulation or coercion.

3. Receive services in a confidential environment that supports her right to make her own decisions regarding her pregnancy through free and candid communication.

4. Be respected enough to make a decision that is right for her by receiving a non-biased presentation of all her pregnancy-related options.

5. Receive comprehensive information about her current medical status, including information about the nature and physiology of her current pregnancy.

6. Access objective information about all of her legal options related to pregnancy and pregnancy termination.

7. Receive services from an organization that has written documentation of all services and information provided, to insure that every patient receives the same objective information delivered with the same standard of excellence.

8. Receive services from an organization that uses a written verification process that services have been provided according to written protocol per patient.

9. Fully understand how a clinician stands to financially profit from any particular pregnancy decision a woman may choose to make at that organization.

10. Receive standardized medical services by clinicians held accountable to follow current medical standards of practice designed to insure that all services and information are delivered ethically and objectively.

11. Assurance of high-quality medical follow-up care provided by or arranged by the clinician responsible for the initial delivery of service.

12. Access to ongoing, long-term community support should she choose to carry the pregnancy to full-term.

Patient Responsibilities

1. Patient is responsible for providing all pertinent and accurate health history, personal circumstances, and belief information to the clinician.

2. Patient is responsible to participate in determining her treatment plan.

3. Patient is responsible to follow prescribed treatment agreed upon with clinician.

4. Patient is responsible to understand his/her rights.

5. Patient is responsible to communicate suggestions, complaints, and grievances using an exit survey process, completed at the end of each appointment.

I, _____, understand my rights and responsibilities.

Signature:_____Date:_____

4. Suggested Case Process for Protecting Patient Facing Unplanned Pregnancy

Service Steps in Chronological Order as Experienced by Patient:

1. Marketing (ethical advertising and awareness of services)

    a. Set appropriate expectations through education oriented messages

2. Contextualized Contact Initiation

    a. Set expectations for services (education oriented)

    b. Set initial appointment

    c. Appointment confirmation

    d. Affirm and reaffirm relevance of services to her condition

    e. Knowledge acquisition for organization about patient and vice versa

3. Intake (Start of official patient/clinician relationship)

    a. Convey rights and responsibilities of patient and clinician

    b. Situational Assessment (coercive pressure identification, determine patient values, beliefs, etc.)

4. Data Collection/Diagnostic Cycle (refer for all treatments that are medically indicated)

    a. Patient presentation (presumptive diagnosis of pregnancy begins)

    b. On-site Pregnancy Test

    c. Physical Exam with Health History including name of primary clinician

    d. Diagnostic ultrasound

    e. STD Testing if indicated

5. Solve (treatment, mother and baby both viable patients consistent with either clinician right of conscience or patient belief)

    a. Options presentation (Patient education including definitions)

    b. Determination of Surrogacy (parent to child consistent with patient beliefs)

    c. Personalized Solutions addressing obstacles to treatment plan consistent with patient

    d. Patient Intention/engagement/plan of care including referral to primary clinician

6. Ensure Continuity of Care (follow-up and service referral)

B. Sample Documentation for Pertinent Ethical Standards

1. Helpline Script

If caller asks to make an appointment and does not indicate what type of appointment they are looking for, ask: "Are you looking for Pregnancy testing or STD testing?" They will most likely give you a clear answer that will indicate pregnancy (or possibly abortion/term), STD testing, or a service we don't provide. If patient is not clear about intention ask "Are you considering termination with this pregnancy at an early, yet appropriate time in the call."

If caller is obviously abortion minded based on what she says:

"A lot of our patients feel a sense of urgency to take care of this quickly, and a little overwhelmed, but you have some time.

There are three medical issues that every woman needs to know before determining the outcome of her pregnancy. So first things first...

1.) "We need to find out if you're really pregnant."
"31% of pregnancies end on their own. Since a positive pregnancy test cannot medically confirm that you are pregnant we need to do **an ultrasound to confirm that you're really pregnant**. Let's schedule you for an appt."

2.) " Next, once your pregnancy is confirmed we need to find out exactly how far along you are."
"Knowing exactly how far along you are determines what type of termination procedure you could get **and how much it will cost you**. This is done using an ultrasound scan. Let's schedule you for an appointment to meet with a nurse and have an ultra sound to confirm your pregnancy and see how far along you are. Our next available time is..."

3.) Finally, before you schedule a termination procedure, you need to have STD testing.
If patient is Abortion Minded and has not scheduled:
"Before I let you go you may want to consider **a pre-termination evaluation that** includes STD testing and treatment so that we can help you **protect your health for a future pregnancy**. It is important that you have STD testing to make sure you don't have Chlamydia or Gonorrhea. If you have a termination procedure with an untreated STD, it can increase your risk of contracting Pelvic Inflammatory Disease by 25%. My next available appointment is _____. Would that time work for you?"

[If patient is not clearly abortion minded, but still has not scheduled, we should replace "pre-termination evaluation" with "appointment"]

If patient (who has not already received all of our services somewhere else) does not schedule- usually b/c they're looking for a place that does the termination procedure say:

"We do not do the termination procedures or refer for them because we are a non-profit organization specializing in objective information and service delivery that does not make any money from your decision. But, we provide the pre-termination evaluation so that we can help you **protect your health for a future pregnancy**. Are you sure you don't want to come in on - _____ for that appointment?"

Conclusion:

"At your appointment, you'll meet **your nurse** who will do a pregnancy test, and if that's positive, an ultrasound, as well as STD testing. She will answer any medical questions you may have, including questions about abortion procedures, in addition to reviewing all of your pregnancy options and resources. Do you have any questions? **If something changes with your schedule or your pregnancy, Will you please call us if you can not make it to your appointment? (Pause and wait for response) Thank you, that enables us to offer it to someone else who is waiting." (Ok, and if something does change with your pregnancy it is still valuable for you to come for STD testing to protect your health for future pregnancy.**

Typical questions:
  Cost:
  - "Our services would cost you $350.00, but we are a non-profit organization whose generous donors have paid that fee on your behalf. Will you please call us if you cannot make it to your appointment?" (Pause and wait for response) Thank you, that enables us to offer that appointment to someone else who is waiting."

  -
  "So you don't actually do abortions/terminations"
  -"We do not do termination procedures or refer for them because we are a non-profit organization that does not make any money from your decision, but we provide the pre-termination evaluation so that we can help you **protect your health for a future pregnancy**, during and after that procedure."

  If patient asks question about morning after pill, or specific medical questions:

  "I'm sorry, I am not a medical professional so it is unlawful for me to answer those questions, but our nurses are very capable and you may ask them any medical questions you have when you meet with them during your appointment. Our next available appointment is... would that work for you?"

2. Waiting Room Brochure

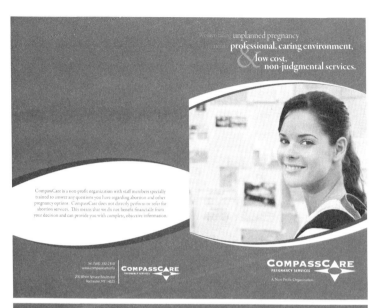

unplanned pregnancy
professional, caring environment,
& low cost,
non-judgmental services.

CompassCare is a non-profit organization with staff members specially trained to answer any questions you have regarding abortion and other pregnancy options. CompassCare does not directly perform or refer for abortion services. This means that we do not benefit financially from your decision and can provide you with complete, objective information.

Tel. (585) 232-2350
www.compasscare.info
210 White Spruce Boulevard
Rochester, NY 14623

COMPASSCARE
PREGNANCY SERVICES

COMPASSCARE
PREGNANCY SERVICES
A Non-Profit Organization

ABOUT COMPASSCARE

CompassCare understands that a woman experiencing an unplanned pregnancy or Sexually Transmitted Infection (STI) may face some of the most difficult decisions she will ever make. CompassCare specializes in helping women get the information they need so they can make those decisions with confidence.

When asked why they would refer a friend to CompassCare, patients said this:

- *"I felt very comfortable; the nurse and advocate genuinely cared about my feelings."*
- *"Very helpful, friendly environment, that makes you as a person feel comfortable."*
- *"Because now I have hope."*

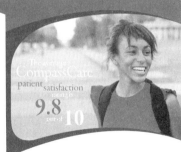

The average CompassCare patient satisfaction rating is

9.8 out of **10**

EVERY WOMAN NEEDS TO HAVE ANSWERS TO THREE BASIC QUESTIONS WHEN CONSIDERING HER PREGNANCY OPTIONS

1. *Am I really pregnant?*

   It is possible to have a positive pregnancy test and not have a viable pregnancy.

2. *If I am pregnant, how far along am I (gestational age)?*

   Gestational age determines what type of abortion procedure a patient would be eligible to receive. Abortion procedures have different costs and side effects.

3. *Is it important to know if I have a Sexually Transmitted Infection (STI)?*

   A woman with a common STI such as chlamydia, if left untreated prior to pregnancy termination, puts her future reproductive health at risk due to increased risk of infection complications.

COMPASSCARE PROVIDES MEDICAL SERVICES SUCH AS:

- Pregnancy testing
- Ultrasound exams, providing earliest pregnancy confirmation available
- Selected STI screening
- Pregnancy options consultation
- Personalized Solutions Assessments (PSA) providing a roadmap of community referrals and helpful information
- Follow up throughout your decision-making process
- Reproductive health seminars

91

3. Print Out

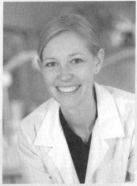

4. Patient Intake Form

Situational Assessment:

Reason for Today's Visit

_____

_____

Pregnancy Test Information

1st Day of Last Period (LMP) _____   Date PT Taken _____

Weeks of Gestation from LMP _____   ❑ Home   ❑ Positive

Expected Due Date from LMP _____   ❑ Dr's Ofc   ❑ Negative

Intention to Carry

How do you feel about potentially being pregnant? _____

_____

If your test is positive, what are your intentions?

❑ Parent   ❑ Abort   ❑ Adopt   ❑ Undecided

Support System Review

What is the father of the baby's First Name?

Does the father of the baby know you are here today?   ❑ Yes ❑ No

Did the father of the baby come here with you today?   ❑ Yes ❑ No

What decision would the father of the baby like you to make
regarding the outcome of your pregnancy?   _____

Who will support you if you choose to continue your
pregnancy?   _____

Who will support you if you decide not to continue your
pregnancy?   _____

Options Presentation

Complete Presentation	Option	Patient's Response
❑	Abortion	_____
❑	Adoption	_____
❑	Parenting	_____

☐ Support System Review using PSA
☐ Ultrasound Exam/Medical Exam Report
☐ Delivery of Personalized Solutions Assessment

Abortion Vulnerability Rating

	Risk Factors	Explain Patient Details (Complete applicable lines)
❏	Still in school (H.S./college/grad)	
❏	Between 17 and 26 years old	
❏	Father of baby in favor of abortion	
❏	Parents in favor of abortion	
❏	History of abortion	
❏	Financial pressure	
❏	Single	
❏	Patient states intention to abort	
	(AM, *regardless of other risk factors*)	

_____ =

Total   Abortion Vulnerability   *Key: 0 = CTT, 1-3 = AV, 4-7 = AM*

Church Background
Religious Affiliation _____

Are you currently active in a church? ❏ Yes ❏ No

Name of Church _____

Evangelism Summary
❏ Patient claims to already be a Christian

❏ I gave a complete/thorough presentation of the Gospel

Patient's response to Gospel presentation: _____

If the patient did not respond positively what is preventing her from receiving Christ?

❏ Patient accepted Christ

❏ We had a Christ–centered religious discussion, but I did not present the Gospel

I did not give a complete presentation because: _____

Closing Summary:

1. "Is there any other information you feel you need to make an informed decision?"

2. "Having received your Personalized Solutions Assessment and all the other information from CompassCare today, what do you think the outcome of your pregnancy will be?"

     ❏ Parent   ❏ Abort   ❏ Adopt   ❏ Undecided

Other Notes:

5. Personalized Solutions Assessment

Patient's Name _____

Nurse's Name _____

Insurance/Financial Assistance
- ❑ Prenatal Care Assistance Program (PCAP)
  1-800-552-5006
- ❑ Fidelis Health Care
  Referral form at CompassCare
- ❑ Women, Infant, Children (WIC)
  585-753-4942

Doctors
- ❑ Dr. Waldemar Klimek, FACOG
  Penfield OB/GYN
  (Accepts Blue Choice Option)
  43 Willow Pond Way, Suite 200
  Penfield, NY 14526
  585.377.5420
  (has other offices in Irondequoit and Farmington)

- ❑ Dr. Katherine Lammers, FACOG
  Greece Obstetrics & Gynecology
  (Accepts Blue Choice Option)
  120 Erie Canal Drive, Suite 200
  Rochester, NY 14626
  585-225-6680

- ❑ Dr. Sareena Fazili, MD, FACOG
  Unity OB/GYN at Parkway
  (Accepts Medicaid)
  500 Island Cottage Rd.
  Rochester, NY 14612
  585-368-6040

- ❑ Dr. Julius Avorkliyah, MD, FACOG
  Unity OB/GYN at West Main
  (Accepts Medicaid)
  819 West Main St.
  Rochester, NY 14611
  585-235-4860

General Health
- ❑ NY State Smoker's Quit Line
  1-866-NY-QUITS

Education & Financial Aid
- ❑ Roberts Wesleyan College
  Faith Haven Single Moms Scholarship
  585-594-6636
- ❑ www.GED-online.co

Financial Counseling
- ❑ Joshua A. Barrett
  Financial Advisor
  www.barrettcm.com/josh@barrettcm.com
  585-383-5556

Pediatricians
- ❑ Dr. Timothy Hessert 585-227-7600
- ❑ Genesis Pediatrics 585-426-4100

Material Assistance
- ❑ Hope Lutheran Church, call 723-4673 M-F
  (identify yourself as our patient)
- ❑ Angel Care at Guardian Angels Church
  Requires CC Nurse referral at 1-2 mo. before due date
  585-321-0236
- ❑ Catholic Family Center
  585-232-2050
  Walk-In hours: M-F 9am-12pm, 1pm-2pm

Adoption
- ❑ Catholic Family Services 585-262-7078
- ❑ Bethany Christian Services 585-288-6760
  Contact: Jennifer Anderson, MSW

Church Referral

_____

_____

_____

_____

Return Appointment Date:

Return Appointment Time:

6. Patient Bill of Rights

Bill of Rights for
Women Facing Unintended Pregnancy

A Woman Facing Unintended Pregnancy Has The Right To:

1. Receive services in a non-judgmental, caring environment committed to maintaining confidentiality of patient records except where required by law.

2. Receive professional medical services from organizations committed to integrity, free from manipulation or coercion.

3. Receive services in a confidential environment that supports her right to make her own decisions regarding her pregnancy.

4. Be respected enough to make a decision that is right for her by receiving a non-biased presentation of all her pregnancy-related options.

5. Receive comprehensive information about her current medical status, including information about the nature and physiology of her current pregnancy.

6. Access objective information about all of her legal options related to pregnancy and pregnancy termination.

7. Receive services from an organization that has written documentation of all services and information provided, to insure that every patient receives the same objective information delivered with the same standard of excellence.

8. Receive services from an organization that uses a written verification process that services have been provided according to written protocol on a per-patient basis.

9. Fully understand how an organization stands to financially profit from any particular pregnancy decision a woman may choose to make at that organization.

10. Receive standardized medical services by organizations held accountable to follow protocols designed to insure that all services and information are delivered ethically and objectively.

11. Assurance of high quality medical follow-up care provided by or arranged by the physician responsible for the initial delivery of service.

12. Access to ongoing, long-term community support should she choose to carry the pregnancy to full-term.

Patient Responsibilities

1. Patient is responsible for providing all pertinent and accurate health history information to provider.
2. Patient is responsible to participate in determining her treatment plan.
3. Patient is responsible to follow prescribed treatment agreed upon with provider.
4. Patient is responsible to understand his/her rights.
5. Patient is responsible to communicate suggestions, complaints, grievances using an exit survey process, completed at the end of each appointment.

I, _____, understand my rights and responsibilities.
   (Print Name)

Signature:_____   Date:_____

---

7. Waiver of Patient Right to Informed Consent

Caution on the Use of Waiver

In most cases the introduction of this Waiver by a medical provider without the request of a patient represents a conflict of interest. The patient's right to waive informed consent should only be presented by the provider when requested by the patient or indicated by statements such as: 'I don't want to know;' 'I can't make this decision;' 'Do whatever you think is best;' etc.

Part 1 – Understanding of Rights

I. I have had a discussion with my medical provider regarding the nature and significance of my right to informed consent and that it DOES NOT INCLUDE a waiver of the provider's right to refuse treatment.

Circle: YES   NO   Initial:_____

I fully understand that:

> A. As an autonomous, self-determining individual I have a right to informed consent.
>
> Circle: YES   NO   Initial:_____
>
> B. My medical provider is legally and ethically obligated to provide me with information regarding (1) the nature of my current condition and diagnosis with pertinent test results, (2) the general nature of all available treatment options, and (3) the risks, side-effects, and prospects of success of each treatment (including non-treatment).
>
> Circle: YES   NO   Initial:_____
>
> C. It is my privilege and responsibility to make all final decisions regarding the treatment of my own person, or the person to whom I am a surrogate.
>
> Circle: YES   NO   Initial:_____

II. I have had a discussion with my medical provider regarding the nature and significance of my right to waive informed consent releasing my medical provider from the obligation to communicate pertinent information about my condition or treatment options.

Circle: YES   NO   Initial:_____

I fully understand that:

> A. I can choose to give up my right to information regarding my condition and available treatment options with their risks.
>
> Circle: YES   NO   Initial:_____

B. If I choose to waive my right to information, subsequent treatments administered by my medical professional may involve known risks and dangers of serious bodily injury, including permanent disability, infertility, paralysis and death, of which I WILL NOT BE MADE AWARE.

Circle: YES   NO   Initial:_____

C. I can choose to give up my right to decide which treatment option to pursue for my current condition, forfeiting that decision-making power to my medical professional.

Circle: YES   NO   Initial:_____

D. If I choose to waive my right to decide, the treatment course which my medical provider chooses may NOT be that which I would have chosen, and may NOT take into account my beliefs, values or future health goals.

Circle: YES   NO   Initial:_____

_____
Patient's Name Printed

_____   _____   _____
Patient's Signature   Date   Time

_____   _____   _____
Medical Provider's Signature   Date   Time

_____   _____   _____
Signature of Witness   Date   Time

Part 2 –Affirmation of Waiver

III. I have completed Part 1 of this Waiver with my medical provider; it has been signed and witnessed.

Circle: YES   NO   Initial:_____

IV. Since this waiver is an act of self-determination by nature I understand that I maintain my right to refuse treatment and that I can suspend this waiver verbally or in writing at any time before, during, or after treatment and all ethical obligations for provider communication subsequent to that point apply.

Circle: YES   NO   Initial:_____

V. I understand that BY SIGNING THIS WAIVER I GIVE UP SUBSTANTIAL RIGHTS, and I confirm that I am under no coercion from family, peers or medical providers; and that I am not under emotional, physical, psychological duress or haste. I am of sound mind and under no sedation whatsoever. I do not feel pressured by my medical provider or any other party to sign this Waiver, but have asked do so of my own free will.

Circle: YES   NO   Initial:_____

VI. In consideration of my personal autonomy and self-determination, I understand that I am entitled to formal control over final decisions regarding my health and active participation in the decision-making process, but I CHOOSE INSTEAD TO FORFEIT MY RIGHT to:

(Check and initial the rights you wish to waive.)

  ☐ _____ RECEIVE INFORMATION regarding:

    ☐_____ The nature of my current condition and diagnosis, with pertinent test results

    ☐_____ The known risks and side-effects of each treatment option.

    ☐_____ The prospects of success of each treatment option.

    ☐_____ My prognosis without treatment.

  ☐ _____ DECIDE which treatment course to pursue.

_____
Patient's Name Printed

_____   _____   _____
Patient's Signature   Date   Time

_____   _____   _____
Medical Provider's Signature   Date   Time

_____   _____   _____
Signature of Witness   Date   Time

99

8. Abortion Information Brochure

Protect Your Health

COMPASSCARE
www.compasscare.info

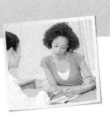

Future Pregnancy Complications

Abortion is associated with an increased risk of low birth weight and preterm birth. The risk increases with each additional abortion. There is also an increase in infertility rates among women who have had previous abortions.

Breast Cancer

Studies show that abortion may increase a woman's risk of breast cancer. A recent analysis revealed a 44% increased risk of breast cancer among women who had at least one induced abortion. The risk increased significantly for those who had two or more abortions.

STDs & Pelvic Inflammatory Disease (PID)

There is a high prevalence rate of Chlamydia and Gonorrhea among women presenting for abortion. Women with an untreated chlamydial infection at the time of abortion have a 72% risk of developing PID.

Mental Health

Women who had an abortion experienced an 81% increased risk of mental health problems, and nearly 10% of the incidence of mental health problems was shown to be attributable to abortion.

Abortion

Research shows that most women want to be informed of risks and treatment alternatives, prior to making their decision.

Costs
Procedures
Development
Health Risks

Within 10 weeks of LMP*
Last Menstrual Period
Chemical Abortion: Mifeprex & Misoprostol
Cost: $200-$800

The FDA approved regimen for a chemical abortion is a two-visit process using two different drugs:

- Mifeprex is given orally during the first office visit. (200 mg) Mifeprex blocks progesterone from sustaining the pregnancy thereby ending the life of the baby.
- Misoprostol is given inside the cheek (800 mcg) 24-48 hours later. This drug will cause contractions to expel the baby's remains. This does not take place at the medical office and may occur within a few hours or up to two weeks after taking the misoprostol.
- A physical exam should be given 7-14 days later to ensure the abortion is complete and that there are no immediate complications.

Risks & Side Effects

- Unsuccessful up to 10% of the time.
- Cramping, nausea, vomiting, diarrhea, heavy bleeding, infection and in rare cases, death.
- Not advised for women who have anemia, bleeding disorders, liver or kidney disease, seizure disorder, acute inflammatory bowel disease, use an IUD, or are unable to return for a follow-up visit.

Fetal Development (Weeks 4-8)

- Nerves, brain and spinal cord begin to develop
- Heart begins to beat
- Eyes, arms, legs, lungs and stomach begin to form
- Genitals form
- All organs are present by week 8

Abortion Pill Reversal
There is a 64%-68% chance of continuing a healthy pregnancy if therapy is started within 72 hours of taking Mifeprex. Call 877-558-0333 or visit abortionpillreversal.com

---

6-16 Weeks After LMP
Surgical Abortion: Suction/Vacuum Aspiration
Cost: $600-$1600

- Patient will lie on her back with feet in stirrups and a speculum is inserted to open the vagina.
- A local anesthetic is administered to her cervix. Then, a tenaculum is used to hold the cervix in place so that it can be dilated by cone-shaped rods.
- When the cervix is wide enough, a cannula is inserted into the uterus to suction out the baby and placenta.
- The procedure usually takes 10-15 minutes with a recovery period of up to 5 hours.
- Based upon the size of the baby, a D&C may also be required, particularly in the second trimester, the provider will use a long loop-shaped knife called a curette to scrape the lining, placenta and baby away from the uterus.

Risks & Side Effects

- Abdominal pain, nausea, sweating, and feeling faint.
- Less frequent side effects include possible heavy or prolonged bleeding, blood clots, damage to the cervix and perforation of the uterus.
- Infection due to retained remains of the baby and related tissues, an STD, or bacteria being introduced to the uterus can cause fever, pain, abdominal tenderness, scarring, infertility and in rare cases, death.

Fetal Development (Weeks 9-16)

- Organs begin functioning
- Skin and fingerprints begin to form
- Baby moves. Kicks and begins sucking thumb

In the medical community choice is referred to as patient autonomy which means you have the right to say "NO" to any medical procedure. If you feel abortion is your only option, you have no freedom of choice.

17-24 Weeks After LMP
Late-Term Surgical Abortion: Dilation & Evacuation
Cost: $1500-$2500

- In most cases, 24 hours prior to the actual procedure, the abortion provider will insert laminaria or a synthetic dilator inside the cervix.
- At the time of the procedure, cone-shaped rods of increasing size are used to continue the dilation process.
- Depending upon gestational age, some providers may deliver a shot with a long needle through the patient's abdomen to cause the baby to die before the procedure begins.
- A cannula is inserted to begin removing the baby from the lining, and the lining is scraped with a curette to remove any residual fetal parts.
- For larger babies, forceps may be used to remove larger parts and some providers prefer to crush the skull for easier extraction.
- The procedure normally takes about 30 minutes, with extended recovery time.

Late-term abortion procedures become increasingly complex and carry more significant risks as the size of the baby increases.

Risks & Side Effects

- Abdominal pain, bleeding, and nausea may occur for two weeks following the procedure.
- Infection due to retained remains of the baby and related tissues, an STD, or bacteria can cause fever, pain, abdominal tenderness, scarring and in some cases, death.
- Although rare, additional risks related to D&E are damage to the uterine lining or cervix, perforation of the uterus, infertility, infection and blood clots.

Fetal Development (Weeks 17-24)

- The five senses develop
- Facial features become distinct
- Mother feels movement more strongly
- It is possible that the fetus can feel pain

100

9. Medical Exam Report

CompassCare

Medical Exam Report: Ultrasound

Name _____ DOB ____ / ____ / ____ Ultrasound # _____

Orders:
- ❏ Urine Pregnancy Testing   Results + / –   Nurse Initials _____
- ❏ Gonorrhea and Chlamydia Testing
- ❏ Vitamin Angels Women's Prenatal Vit/Min Supplement   Lot Number: 3H7126071277-180   Exp. Date 08/30/2016

_____ CompassCare Medical Services Director: _Dr. Katherine Lammers, MD_ x _____

_____ Name of follow-up physician: _____

_____ pt was referred to _____ Hospital ED via ambulance

Signature of nurse completing test _____ Date _____

Ultrasound not performed:
- ❏ **Negative Test**
- ❏ **Patient Refused**
- ❏ **Bleeding/Increased pain**
- ❏ **Too early; GA by LMP:** ____ weeks, ____ days

Ultrasound Exam Report:
- ❏ Please do limited OB ultrasound, indication   Confirmation of intrauterine pregnancy and determination of gestational age

    X _____ MD _____ / ____ / ____

Date of U/S _____ Abdominal _____ Transvaginal _____

FHR _____ Fetal number _____

GS: _____ cm x _____ cm x _____ cm CRL: _____ cm BPD: _____ cm FL: _____ cm

LMP ____ / ____ / ____

| | | | | | | |
Gestational Age by LMP _____ weeks _____ days EDC by LMP _____ / ____ / ____

Gestational Age by U/S _____ weeks _____ days EDC by U/S ____ / ____ / ____

Ultrasound Notes:

- ❏ **STD Testing requested**

_____ pt was given "So, You're Pregnant" brochure

_____ pt was given "Unable To Confirm Viability Of Pregnancy" brochure

_____ pt to follow up for repeat ultrasound/STD results   Date _____ Time _____ AM / PM

Signature of RN/LPN/RDMS completing exam _____ RN/LPN/RDMS Date _____

Physician signature for review of the ultrasound _____ Date _____

Presumptive Diagnosis of Pregnancy shall be provided for patients who meet the following criteria:
- ❏ Positive in-house urine pregnancy test
- ❏ Presence of gestational sac in uterus
- ❏ Presence of fetal pole in uterus
- ❏ Presence of fetal heart sounds

If all four of the above criteria are met upon patient exam, presumptive diagnosis may be communicated by the RN to the patient, confirming pregnancy. Review gestational age per ultrasound and appropriate fetal development.

- ❏ Confirmed with patient Date:_____ Signature of nurse:_____

Medical Director signature for final review of the chart _____ Date _____

10. Initial Visit Health Questionnaire

Name:_____ DOB:_____

Gender: ☐ Male ☐ Female   ☐ STD Pt   ☐ Pregnancy Pt

Chief Complaint _____

STD Patients Only:

 # Sexual Partners   Past 90 Days _____

 # Times You've Had Sex   Past 90 Days _____

Have you ever:

	Given		Received	
Anal Sex?		M		M / F
Vaginal Sex?		M		F
Oral Sex?		M / F		M / F

Do you have any of the following:

Sore throat?	Y / N	Frequent urination?	Y / N
Genital pain?	Y / N	Pain/Burning with urination?	Y / N
Abnormal discharge/odor?	Y / N	Blood in urine?	Y / N

ALL PATIENTS:

When was your last STD test?   ☐ Never   Date _____

Have you had any sexual
exposure to a person with a   If yes, when
known STD?   Y / N   and to what?   Date _____

Have you ever had a STD? Y / N   If yes, when?   Date _____

☐ HIV   ☐ Hepatitis (A / B / C)   ☐ Chlamydia   ☐ Gonorrhea

☐ Syphilis   ☐ Genital Warts   ☐ Herpes   ☐ Other

Do you use any of the following: **If Yes, please specify:**

Over the Counter or Prescription Medications?   Y / N

Other Drugs?   Y / N

Cigarettes?   Y / N

Alcohol?   Y / N

Are you allergic to latex?   Y / N

Are you allergic to any foods or medications?   Y / N
(If yes, please list medication and reaction)

Any other health conditions/symptoms/concerns?

Pregnancy and Female STD Patients Only:
OB/GYN history
How many times have you:

Been pregnant _____   Delivered how many children _____   Delivered premature, before 37 wks _____

Miscarried _____   Ectopic pregnancy _____   Had an abortion _____

If Yes to abortion:

❑ Medical   ❑ Surgical   Date: _____   How far along? _____

Have you ever had:
Cesarean section?   Y / N
Infertility?   Y / N
Other problems with pregnancy?   Y / N
An abnormal PAP smear?   Y / N
Date of last PAP:
Name of OB/GYN Physician: _____

Current Health History
When was the first day of your last period?   _____

Was it normal or different from usual?   ❑ Normal   ❑ Abnormal

Are your periods regular?   ❑ Yes   ❑ No   How often do you have a period?   Every _____ days

What kind of birth control have you been using, if any?   _____

When did you last use any hormonal birth control?   _____

Do you or have you had any of the following?

Abdominal pain/cramps:	Y / N	Nausea:		Y / N
If yes- greater than your period:	Y / N	Vomiting:		Y / N
❑ Consistent ❑ Intermittent		Breast tenderness:		Y / N
Vaginal bleeding/spotting:	Y / N	Family History of Breast Cancer		Y / N
Vaginal discharge:	Y / N			
If yes – Odor?	Y / N			
Color?	Y / N			

103

11. Excerpt from the CompassCare STD Testing and Treatment Process

Step:	**#9- Physical Exam and Blood Draw (15 min)** • RN performs physical exam (using Male and Female Scripts) • RN draws blood • RN discusses risks of partner variation and frequency for STD and unplanned pregnancy (Education review) • In-House labs performed by RN following PE (wet preps) • Swabs prepared for shipment to CDD
Owner:	Staff Nurse
Location:	Exam room (equipped with Ultrasound machine for pregnant patients as well as exam table and various supplies needed)

Scripts:	☐ Physical Exam:
	  • **"I will be obtaining several samples, including a swab of your cervix, your rectum and your throat** [state only those indicated during history]. **I will also be looking for other symptoms that may indicate a problem."**
	  ☐ **"I will step out, so you can get undressed from the waist down. You can cover up with this drape sheet. I'll come back in when you're ready."** PE script as determined by Dr. Davey, training
	  ▪ Script for abnormal PE:
	    • **"I'm not seeing what I would expect to see in your exam. Diagnosing abnormalities is outside the scope of my practice, so you need to be seen by a physician immediately."**
	☐ Transition to Blood Draw/Education "Quiz"
	  • **"I will step out so you can get dressed again. When I come back, I'll do your blood draw."**
	☐ Education Review (during blood draw):
	  • **"I've got a little quiz for you. What are two ways you can decrease your risk for STDs and unplanned pregnancy?"** *[Answer: By decreasing your number of sexual partners, and if you have more than one partner, decreasing the number of times you have sex with all of them. This decreases the number of times you're exposed to STDs.]*
	• **Transition to lab work/Introduce Education:**
	  • **"I need to look at your samples under the microscope to see if you have any positive results that we can treat today. While I'm gone, you can think about these three questions and write down some answers if you'd like. We'll talk more about that when I return with your results."**

Forms:	*Physical Exam Report*
Policies:	PHYSICAL EXAMINATION POLICY EDUCATION POLICY
Add'l Print Materials:	
Notes:	Male: Use Male PE guide

Step:	# #10- STD Results & Education (10 mins) • Review results of PE including any positive results (disease specific brochure based on diagnosis) • Review Education Worksheet • Discuss benefits and risks of current sexual health decisions in context of goals stated by patient
Owner:	Staff Nurse
Location:	Exam room

Scripts:	☐ Review PE, wet prep results with patient:
	   ○ Negative results:
	     ■ **"Our lab tests and physical exam did not detect any STDs today. But, there are still some STDs that can only be determined with blood work. You should not have any sexual contact with anyone until you receive those results. Those results will be available in about three business days. I'll discuss how you can get your results in just a moment."**
	   ○ Positive results:
	     ■ **"Our lab tests [AND/OR] physical exam detected [STD]. [AND/OR] Your health history [also] indicates that you may have Chlamydia/ Gonorrhea. You will receive treatment for that today. There are still some STDs that can only be determined with blood work. You should not have any sexual contact with anyone until you receive those results. Those results will be available in about three business days. I'll discuss how you can get your results in just a moment."**
	☐ Brochures serve as scripts for Education
	   ☐ Education Script:
	     ■ **"Did you have a chance to think about some of your goals, and how your sexual health decisions are related to them?"**
	   • Review patient's responses, and engage patient with both positive aspects and negative aspects of sexual health decisions.
	        ○ **"What are some of your goals?"**
	        ○ **"How are your sexual health decisions helping you reach those goals?"**
	        ○ **"How are they hindering you from reaching your goals?"**
	   • Identify one of the patient's goals and discuss positive and negative results of their decision directly related with that goal.
	   • If a patient states a positive aspect that is in fact not healthy or beneficial to him/her, redirect him/her to another positive point that you can then affirm with him/her.
	   •
	   • You can suggest some of the following goals if patient does not have any:
	     ○ Get married
	     ○ Have children
	     ○ Finish school
	     ○ Start a career (What field?)
	     ○ Travel
	   • You can suggest some of the following positives if patient does not have any:
	     ○ Looking for the right guy/girl
	     ○ Learning what I want in a relationship
	     ○ It's fun
	     ○ Get to know someone better
	   • You can suggest some of the following negatives if patient does not have any:

Forms:	
Policies:	REPORTING OF STD AND HIV TEST RESULTS TO PATIENTS AND PARTNERS STD EDUCATION STANDING ORDERS FOR STD TESTING AND TREATMENT
Add'l Print Materials:	• Friend Referral card • Pregnancy test given to negative test patients • Partner Chart
Notes:	

Step:	**#11-STD Treatment (8 mins)**
	• RN explains disease specific treatment (using *Drug Fact Sheet*)
	• RN administers treatment and documents on *STD Panel Form*
	• RN has patient choose results notification method, and sign *Results Consent Form*
Owner:	Staff Nurse
Location:	Exam room
Scripts:	▢ Choosing results notification method:
	• **"We can email your test results to you, along with instructions for obtaining any necessary treatment or follow-up. If you don't have an email address or you don't want to provide it to us, you can also make an appointment to receive your results in person."**
	• RN will review *Results Consent* and have patient initial beside choice and sign.
	• If patient needs to schedule a return appt before leaving, nurse will write timeframe on PSA and Clinical Coordinator will schedule at Check-out.
Forms:	• *Drug Fact Sheets*
	• *Results Consent Form*
	• *STD Panel Form*
Policies:	ALL DISEASE-SPECIFIC POLICIES
	MEDICATION STORAGE AND DISPENSATION POLICY
Add'l Print Materials:	
Notes:	

107

12. Confirmation of Pregnancy Policy

POLICY: VERIFICATIONS OF POSITIVE PREGNANCY TESTS
AND CONFIRMATIONS OF PREGNANCY

Verifications of Positive Pregnancy Tests simply verify that the pregnancy test read positive. Nurses may verify positive pregnancy tests. This is different from a Confirmation of Pregnancy that can only be diagnosed by a physician or nurse practitioner after an exam, such as ultrasound.

The CPS shall provide pregnancy documentation to any patient who requests one for the purposes of obtaining pre-natal care. CPS shall not provide pregnancy documentation to patients intending to use the documentation to obtain an abortion or funding for an abortion. This policy shall be addressed in the initial intake sheet so that the patient is aware of the office's policy in this regard.

PROCEDURE:

VERIFICATION OF POSITIVE PREGNANCY TESTS:

1. Verification of Positive Pregnancy Tests may only be provided after a pregnancy test has been supervised by a nurse or other trained personnel and not on the basis of the results of a self-administered test.

2. If the patient has a positive pregnancy test and wants verification, one shall be provided on the "Verification of Positive Pregnancy Test" form. A nurse or other trained staff shall fill out the form, which shall be signed by the nurse pursuant to the Standing Order.

3. A confirmation of pregnancy shall only be provided by physicians or nurse practitioners after examination.

4. The original form shall be given to the patient and a copy will be placed in the patient's medical record.

13. Limitations of Services

Last Name _____ First Name _____ Date _____

- CompassCare is a non-profit organization. All of our services are free, including a urine pregnancy test, ultrasound if that test is positive, and Sexually Transmitted Disease (STD) testing, as well as a situational assessment and personalized pregnancy options consultation provided by a Nurse.

- The medical services are all referrals and are not performed or provided by CompassCare Pregnancy Services but rather by licensed medical professionals. A physician must confirm your pregnancy test with an ultrasound to determine viability.

- Whether the pregnancy or STD test is positive or negative, you should consult with a licensed physician. If you do not have a physician, your Nurse will offer referrals including that for our medical director, Dr. Katherine Lammers.

- Our Nurses are all trained in crisis counseling though not necessarily licensed or degreed personnel. The counseling obtained here is not intended as a substitute for professional counseling.

- All information is kept confidential except if child abuse or other mandated reporting laws apply or if we believe or hear that you are in danger of hurting yourself or others.

- CompassCare does not perform or refer for abortion, which includes not providing confirmation of pregnancy for abortion retention purposes.

- CompassCare does not profit from your decision.

I have read and understood the above and hereby authorize the staff of this office to render whatever services are necessary for my care.

Patient Signature _____ Date _____

Staff Signature _____ Date _____

14. What Can You Expect? Form

□ Initial Appointment (STD Testing or Pregnancy Appointment)
  * You will meet with a Nurse, who will:
    o Review the Reproductive Health Screening that you will be receiving today, including STD and pregnancy testing
    o For female patients only, perform a pregnancy test. If positive,
      * Review all of your pregnancy options, including "Abortion: Procedures, Risks and Side Effects"
      * Perform an ultrasound exam to confirm pregnancy and determine how far along you are
    o For STD Testing patients:
      * Draw some blood and perform a physical exam to complete your STD Screening
      * Report to you some STD results today and, if positive, provide you with the necessary treatment during your appointment
    o Review your health history
    o Answer your medical questions
    o Review your *Personalized Solutions Assessment* and provide any necessary medical referrals
    o Schedule another appointment for you to receive your test results in one week

□ Return Appointment
  * You will meet with a Nurse, who will:
    o Review your health history since your last visit
    o Provide STD test results and any necessary treatment for positive results
    o Repeat a pregnancy test, if necessary. If positive,
      * Review all of your pregnancy options, including "Abortion: Procedures, Risks and Side Effects"
      * Perform an ultrasound exam to confirm pregnancy and determine how far along you are
    o Answer your medical questions
    o Provide any additional referrals you may need

PRIVACY POLICY

CompassCare encourages the support of friends and family during your appointment. Please note that, in an effort to comply with HIPAA Privacy Standards and provide the highest quality of care, your clinical visit must be performed without any guests. However, patients having an ultrasound exam may choose to invite guests to join them for that portion of their visit. CompassCare staff is unable to provide services to patients who choose not to abide by this policy.

I have read and understand the policy described above.

Patient Signature _____ **Date** _____

15. Authorization for Release of Medical Information

Authorization for Release of Health Information (Including Alcohol/Drug Treatment and Mental Health Information) and Confidential HIV/AIDS-related Information

NEW YORK STATE DEPARTMENT OF HEALTH

Patient Name	Date of Birth	Patient Identification Number
Patient Address		

I, or my authorized representative, request that health information regarding my care and treatment be released as set forth on this form. I understand that:

1. This authorization may include disclosure of information relating to ALCOHOL and DRUG TREATMENT, MENTAL HEALTH TREATMENT, and CONFIDENTIAL HIV/AIDS-RELATED INFORMATION only if I place my initials on the appropriate line in Item 8. In the event the health information described below includes any of these types of information, and I initial the line on the box in Item 8, I specifically authorize release of such information to the person(s) indicated in Item 6.

2. With some exceptions, health information once disclosed may be re-disclosed by the recipient. If I am authorizing the release of HIV/AIDS-related, alcohol or drug treatment, or mental health treatment information, the recipient is prohibited from re-disclosing such information or using the disclosed information for any other purpose without my authorization unless permitted to do so under federal or state law. If I experience discrimination because of the release or disclosure of HIV/AIDS-related information, I may contact the New York State Division of Human Rights at 1-888-392-3644. This agency is responsible for protecting my rights.

3. I have the right to revoke this authorization at any time by writing to the provider listed below in Item 5. I understand that I may revoke this authorization except to the extent that action has already been taken based on this authorization.

4. Signing this authorization is voluntary. I understand that generally my treatment, payment, enrollment in a health plan, or eligibility for benefits will not be conditional upon my authorization of this disclosure. However, I do understand that I may be denied treatment in some circumstances if I do not sign this consent.

5. Name and Address of Provider or Entity to Release this Information:

6. Name and Address of Person(s) to Whom this Information Will Be Disclosed:

7. Purpose for Release of Information:

8. Unless previously revoked by me, the specific information below may be disclosed from: _____ INSERT START DATE _____ until _____ INSERT EXPIRATION DATE OR EVENT

☐ All health information (written and oral), except:

For the following to be included, indicate the specific information to be disclosed and initial below.	Information to be Disclosed	Initials
☐ Records from alcohol/drug treatment programs		
☐ Clinical records from mental health programs*		
☐ HIV/AIDS-related Information		

9. If not the patient, name of person signing form:	10. Authority to sign on behalf of patient:

All items on this form have been completed, my questions about this form have been answered and I have been provided a copy of the form.

SIGNATURE OF PATIENT OR REPRESENTATIVE AUTHORIZED BY LAW _____ DATE

Witness Statement/Signature: I have witnessed the execution of this authorization and state that a copy of the signed authorization was provided to the patient and/or the patient's authorized representative.

STAFF PERSON'S NAME AND TITLE _____ SIGNATURE _____ DATE

This form may be used in place of DOH-2557 and has been approved by the NYS Office of Mental Health and NYS Office of Alcoholism and Substance Abuse Services to permit release of health information. However, this form does not require health care providers to release health information. Alcohol/drug treatment-related information or confidential HIV-related information released through this form must be accompanied by the required statements regarding prohibition of re-disclosure.

*Note: Information from mental health clinical records may be released pursuant to this authorization to the parties identified herein who have a demonstrable need for the information, provided that the disclosure will not reasonably be expected to be detrimental to the patient or another person.

DOH-5032 (4/11)

Complete information for each facility/person to be given general medical information and/or HIV-related information. Attach additional sheets as necessary. It is recommended that blank lines be crossed out prior to signing.

Name and address of facility/person to be given general medical and/or HIV-related information:

_____

_____

_____

Reason for release, if other than stated on page 1:

_____

_____

If information to be disclosed to this facility/person is limited, please specify:

_____

_____

Name and address of facility/person to be given general medical and/or HIV-related information:

_____

_____

_____

Reason for release, if other than stated on page 1:

_____

_____

If information to be disclosed to this facility/person is limited, please specify:

_____

_____

The law protects you from HIV related discrimination in housing, employment, health care and other services. For more information call the New York State Division of Human Rights Office of AIDS Discrimination Issues at 1-800-523-2437 or (212) 480-2522 or the New York City Commission on Human Rights at (212) 306-7500. These agencies are responsible for protecting your rights.

My questions about this form have been answered. I know that I do not have to allow release of my medical and/or HIV-related information, and that I can change my mind at any time and revoke my authorization by writing the facility/person obtaining this release. I authorize the facility/person noted on page one to release medical and/or HIV-related information of the person named on page one to the organizations/persons listed.

Signature _____   Date _____
    (Subject of information or legally authorized representative)

If legal representative, indicate relationship to subject: _____

Print Name _____

Client/Patient Number _____

Complete information for each facility/person to be given general medical information and/or HIV-related information.
Attach additional sheets as necessary. Blank lines may be crossed out prior to signing.

Name and address of facility/person to be given general medical and/or HIV-related information:

_____
_____
_____

Reason for release, if other than stated on page 1:

_____
_____

If information to be disclosed to this facility/person is limited, please specify:

_____
_____

Name and address of facility/person to be given general medical and/or HIV-related information:

_____
_____
_____

Reason for release, if other than stated on page 1:

_____
_____

If information to be disclosed to this facility/person is limited, please specify:

_____
_____

Name and address of facility/person to be given general medical and/or HIV-related information:

_____
_____
_____

Reason for release, if other than stated on page 1:

_____
_____

If information to be disclosed to this facility/person is limited, please specify:

_____
_____

If any/all of this page is completed, please sign below:

Signature _____   Date _____

Client/Patient Number _____

DOH-2557 (8/05) p 3 of 3

16. FDA Mifeprex Medication Guide

MEDICATION GUIDE

Mifeprex (MIF-eh-prex) (mifepristone) tablets, for oral use

Read this information carefully before taking Mifeprex and misoprostol. It will help you understand how the treatment works. This Medication Guide does not take the place of talking with your healthcare provider.

What is the most important information I should know about Mifeprex?

What symptoms should I be concerned with? Although cramping and bleeding are an expected part of ending a pregnancy, rarely, serious and potentially life-threatening bleeding, infections, or other problems can occur following a miscarriage, surgical abortion, medical abortion, or childbirth. Seeking medical attention as soon as possible is needed in these circumstances. Serious infection has resulted in death in a very small number of cases. There is no information that use of Mifeprex and misoprostol caused these deaths. If you have any questions, concerns, or problems, or if you are worried about any side effects or symptoms, you should contact your healthcare provider. You can write down your healthcare provider's telephone number here _____.

Be sure to contact your healthcare provider promptly if you have any of the following:

- **Heavy Bleeding.** Contact your healthcare provider right away if you bleed enough to soak through two thick full-size sanitary pads per hour for two consecutive hours or if you are concerned about heavy bleeding. In about 1 out of 100 women, bleeding can be so heavy that it requires a surgical procedure (surgical aspiration or D&C).

- **Abdominal Pain or "Feeling Sick."** If you have abdominal pain or discomfort, or you are "feeling sick," including weakness, nausea, vomiting, or diarrhea, with or without fever, more than 24 hours after taking misoprostol, you should contact your healthcare provider without delay. These symptoms may be a sign of a serious infection or another problem (including an ectopic pregnancy, a pregnancy outside the womb).

- **Fever.** In the days after treatment, if you have a fever of 100.4°F or higher that lasts for more than 4 hours, you should contact your healthcare provider right away. Fever may be a symptom of a serious infection or another problem.

If you cannot reach your healthcare provider, go to the nearest hospital emergency room. Take this Medication Guide with you. When you visit an emergency room or a healthcare provider who did not give you your Mifeprex, you should give them your Medication Guide so that they understand that you are having a medical abortion with Mifeprex.

What to do if you are still pregnant after Mifeprex with misoprostol treatment. If you are still pregnant, your healthcare provider will talk with you about a surgical procedure to end your pregnancy. In many cases, this surgical procedure can be done in the office/clinic. The chance of birth defects if the pregnancy is not ended is unknown.

Talk with your healthcare provider. Before you take Mifeprex, you should read this Medication Guide and you and your healthcare provider should discuss the benefits and risks of your using Mifeprex.

What is Mifeprex?

Mifeprex is used in a regimen with another prescription medicine called misoprostol, to end an early pregnancy. Early pregnancy means it is 70 days (10 weeks) or less since your last menstrual period began. Mifeprex is not approved for ending pregnancies that are further along. Mifeprex blocks a hormone needed for your pregnancy to continue. When you use Mifeprex on Day 1, you also need to take another medicine called misoprostol 24 to 48 hours after you take Mifeprex, to cause the pregnancy to be passed from your uterus.

The pregnancy is likely to be passed from your uterus within 2 to 24 hours after taking Mifeprex and misoprostol. When the pregnancy is passed from the uterus, you will have bleeding and cramping that will likely be heavier than your usual period. About 2 to 7 out of 100 women taking Mifeprex will need a surgical procedure because the pregnancy did not completely pass from the uterus or to stop bleeding.

Who should not take Mifeprex?

Some women should not take Mifeprex. Do not take Mifeprex if you:

- Have a pregnancy that is more than 70 days (10 weeks). Your healthcare provider may do a clinical examination, an ultrasound examination, or other testing to determine how far along you are in pregnancy.

- Are using an IUD (intrauterine device or system). It must be taken out before you take Mifeprex.

- Have been told by your healthcare provider that you have a pregnancy outside the uterus (ectopic pregnancy).

- Have problems with your adrenal glands (chronic adrenal failure).

- Take a medicine to thin your blood.

- Have a bleeding problem.

- Have porphyria.

- Take certain steroid medicines.

- Are allergic to mifepristone, misoprostol, or medicines that contain misoprostol, such as Cytotec or Arthrotec.

Ask your healthcare provider if you are not sure about all your medical conditions before taking this medicine to find out if you can take Mifeprex.

What should I tell my healthcare provider before taking Mifeprex?

Before you take Mifeprex, tell your healthcare provider if you:

- cannot follow-up within approximately 7 to 14 days of your first visit

- are breastfeeding. Mifeprex can pass into your breast milk. The effect of the Mifeprex and misoprostol regimen on the breastfed infant or on milk production is unknown.

- are taking medicines, including prescription and over-the-counter medicines, vitamins, and herbal supplements.
  Mifeprex and certain other medicines may affect each other if they are used together. This can cause side effects.

115

How should I take Mifeprex?

- Mifeprex will be given to you by a healthcare provider in a clinic, medical office, or hospital.

- You and your healthcare provider will plan the most appropriate location for you to take the misoprostol, because it may cause bleeding, cramps, nausea, diarrhea, and other symptoms that usually begin within 2 to 24 hours after taking it.

- Most women will pass the pregnancy within 2 to 24 hours after taking the misoprostol tablets.

Follow the instruction below on how to take Mifeprex and misoprostol:

Mifeprex (1 tablet) orally + misoprostol (4 tablets) buccally

Day 1:

- Take 1 Mifeprex tablet by mouth.

- Your healthcare provider will either give you or prescribe for you 4 misoprostol tablets to take 24 to 48 hours later.

24 to 48 hours after taking Mifeprex:

- Place 2 misoprostol tablets in each cheek pouch (the area between your teeth and cheek - see Figure A) for 30 minutes and then swallow anything left over with a drink of water or another liquid.

- The medicines may not work as well if you take misoprostol sooner than 24 hours after Mifeprex or later than 48 hours after Mifeprex.

- Misoprostol often causes cramps, nausea, diarrhea, and other symptoms. Your healthcare provider may send you home with medicines for these symptoms.

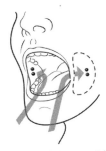

Figure A (2 tablets between your left cheek and gum and 2 tablets between your right cheek and gum).

Follow-up Assessment at Day 7 to 14:

- This follow-up assessment is very important. You must follow-up with your healthcare provider about 7 to 14 days after you have taken Mifeprex to be sure you are well and that you have had bleeding and the pregnancy has passed from your uterus.

- Your healthcare provider will assess whether your pregnancy has passed from your uterus. If your pregnancy continues, the chance that there may be birth defects is unknown. If you are still pregnant, your healthcare provider will talk with you about a surgical procedure to end your pregnancy.

- If your pregnancy has ended, but has not yet completely passed from your uterus, your provider will talk with you about other choices you have, including waiting, taking another dose of misoprostol, or having a surgical procedure to empty your uterus.

When should I begin birth control?

You can become pregnant again right after your pregnancy ends. If you do not want to become pregnant again, start using birth control as soon as your pregnancy ends or before you start having sexual intercourse again.

What should I avoid while taking Mifeprex and misoprostol?

Do not take any other prescription or over-the-counter medicines (including herbal medicines or supplements) at any time during the treatment period without first asking your healthcare provider about them because they may interfere with the treatment. Ask your healthcare provider about what medicines you can take for pain and other side effects.

What are the possible side effects of Mifeprex and misoprostol?

Mifeprex may cause serious side effects. See "What is the most important information I should know about Mifeprex?"

Cramping and bleeding. Cramping and vaginal bleeding are expected with this treatment. Usually, these symptoms mean that the treatment is working. But sometimes you can get cramping and bleeding and still be pregnant. This is why you must follow-up with your healthcare provider approximately 7 to 14 days after taking Mifeprex. See "How should I take Mifeprex?" for more information on your follow-up assessment. If you are not already bleeding after taking Mifeprex, you probably will begin to bleed once you take misoprostol, the medicine you take 24 to 48 hours after Mifeprex. Bleeding or spotting can be expected for an average of 9 to16 days and may last for up to 30 days. Your bleeding may be similar to, or greater than, a normal heavy period. You may see blood clots and tissue. This is an expected part of passing the pregnancy.

The most common side effects of Mifeprex treatment include: nausea, weakness, fever/chills, vomiting, headache, diarrhea and dizziness. Your provider will tell you how to manage any pain or other side effects.These are not all the possible side effects of Mifeprex.

Call your healthcare provider for medical advice about any side effects that bother you or do not go away. You may report side effects to FDA at 1-800-FDA-1088.

General information about the safe and effective use of Mifeprex.

Medicines are sometimes prescribed for purposes other than those listed in a Medication Guide. This Medication Guide summarizes the most important information about Mifeprex. If you would like more information, talk with your healthcare provider. You may ask your healthcare provider for information about Mifeprex that is written for healthcare professionals.

For more information about Mifeprex, go to www.earlyoptionpill.com or call 1-877-4 Early Option (1-877-432-7596).

Manufactured for: *Danco Laboratories, LLC*
P.O. Box 4816
New York, NY 10185
1-877-4 Early Option (1-877-432-7596) www.earlyoptionpill.com

This Medication Guide has been approved by the U.S. Food and Drug Administration.   Approval 3/2016

17. Sample Follow-up Process

Follow Up Process for a Positive Viable Pregnancy

1. Pt. appt: u/s
2. 2nd pt. appt. and/or u/s
3. Dr. Lammers signs **Medical Exam Report**, confirming u/s and viability
4. Call pt.
   a. Up to 3 x's to confirm pregnancy
   b. Document conversation on **Pregnancy Confirmation Form, Patient Contact Form** and at the bottom of the **Medical Exam Report**

   c. If unable to reach pt. after 3 x's
      i. Send certified letter and document on the **Medical Exam Report and the Patient Contact Form.**
      ii. If patient does not respond to certified letter after two weeks, file for final MD signature.
      iii. Once MD gives final signature, stamp it with *Chart Medically Closed* stamp.
      iv. Do not schedule for additional follow up calls
      v. Keep chart open and close after due date with a **Closing Summary Form.**

   d. If able to reach patient and have confirmed pregnancy with her:

      i. Have Dr. Lammers give final signature.
      ii. Once MD gives final signature, stamp it with *Chart Medically Closed* stamp.
      iii. Schedule PR follow up at 4, 8, 16 weeks from initial visit.
      iv. Document calls on **Patient Contact Form** and details of call on **Follow Up Form**
      v. Call patient for final call 4 weeks after due date and document on **Closing Summary Form.**
      vi. File chart for NM to sign.

5. If patient aborts or miscarries, document on **Closing Summary Form.** (Do not use **Follow-Up Form** since a final outcome is known and that call becomes a closing call.)

Follow Up Process for a Negative Test/Non-Viable Pregnancy

1. 2 weeks following the appt.
   a. Call patient one time to follow up and close.
   b. If you reach the patient:
      i. Ask if she got her period. If no, offer another appointment.
      ii. Document on **Negative Test Follow Up** Form and **Closing Summary.**
      iii. File chart for final MD signature.
      iv. After Final MD Signature, stamp to close chart.
   c. If you don't reach the patient:
      i. Document that call was attempted on **Closing Summary.**
      ii. File chart for final MD signature.
      iii. After Final MD Signature, stamp to close chart.
      iv. File chart for NM to sign.

18. Closing Summary Form

Chart Closing Summary Form

Patient Name: _____

Date First Seen: _____   Date of Closing Call: _____

□ Negative Test
Notes: _____

□ Miscarriage
Date of miscarriage: _____

Notes: _____

□ Abortion Performed
Type of abortion: □ Medical   □ Surgical

Date of abortion: _____

Location of abortion: _____

How is patient feeling? _____

How are patient's family/boyfriend relationships? _____

_____

Referrals requested: _____

Post-Abortion Syndrome indicated by patient?   □ Yes   □ No

Interested in Abortion Recovery counseling?   □ Yes   □ No

Notes: _____

□ Child Born
Date of Birth: _____   Gender: □ Male   □ Female

Baby's Name: _____

Weight: _____   Length: _____

Date of baby visit: _____   □ Office Visit   □ Home Visit

□ Unable to Contact

□ Patient Requested No Further Contact

□ Other
Closing Notes: _____

_____

RN Signature: _____ Date: _____

19. Patient Chart Outline

Patient Resources
Closing Summary Form
Patient Contact Form
Photo Release
Patient Follow-up Form
Return Visit Form
Patient Intake Form
Personalized Solutions Assessment
Helpline Intake Form

Medical Services
Pregnancy Confirmation Form
Release of Medical Information
Patient Correspondence
Ultrasound Images
Medical Exam Report
Health Questionnaire
Ultrasound Consent Form
STD Consent Form

20. STD Education Script

20. STD Education Script

STD Education Script:

- "Did you have a chance to think about some of your goals, and how your sexual health decisions are related to them?"
- Review patient's responses, and engage patient with both positive aspects and negative aspects of sexual health decisions.
  - "What are some of your goals?"
  - "How are your sexual health decisions helping you reach those goals?"
  - "How are they hindering you from reaching your goals?"
- Identify one of the patient's goals and discuss positive and negative results of their decision directly related with that goal.
- If a patient states a positive aspect that is in fact not healthy or beneficial to him/her, redirect him/her to another positive point that you can then affirm with him/her.
-
- You can suggest some of the following goals if patient does not have any:
  - Get married
  - Have children
  - Finish school
  - Start a career (What field?)
  - Travel
- You can suggest some of the following positives if patient does not have any:
  - Looking for the right guy/girl
  - Learning what I want in a relationship
  - It's fun
  - Get to know someone better
- You can suggest some of the following negatives if patient does not have any:
  - Put yourself at risk for future reproductive health problems (i.e. PID, HIV)
  - Many STDs have no cure
  - You risk passing them on to another partner
  - Symptoms are often difficult to deal with
  - Unplanned pregnancy is a very difficult situation
- We have already talked about two ways you can decrease your risk of getting a STD or getting pregnant. First, only have sex with one person, who is also only having sex with you. Second, if you do have more than one partner, reduce the number of times you have sex with all of them. This reduces the number of times you are exposed to a STD." [Use *How At Risk Are You*]

"It is important for your partners to get tested, even if all of your results are negative. You can give them this card, and we will make an appointment for them to have the same tests that you've had today." [Give Friend Referral Card]

21. STD Education Worksheet

COMPASSC▲RE

Name_____

What are some of your life goals? (Examples: Get married, have children, get a college degree, become a business owner, etc.)

-
-

-

What are some ways your sexual health decisions are helping you reach these goals?

-
-

-

What are some ways your sexual health decisions are hindering you from reaching those goals?

-
-

-

22. Health Questionnaire Breakdown

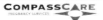

Health Questionnaire Breakdown:

Table of Contents

History of Previous Pregnancies:

It is important to know how many times she has been pregnant before and what the outcome of each pregnancy was. This will give us an idea of how she might decide in this pregnancy, as well as, clue us into any side effects she may be experiencing from a previous abortion.

(Do not shy away from using the word abortion. This is a professional setting and medically we need to know what her history is if we are going to be able to help her today).

It is important to get any information surrounding any previous miscarriages, ectopic pregnancies, and abortions that might be helpful, such as how long ago, how far along was she, what happened, where, who did it, what procedure did she have. *CompassCare can use this information for tracking purposes.*

Normal Menstrual Cycle and Pregnancy:

The textbook menstrual cycle is 28 days in length, with ovulation occurring on or about day 14. The first day of a woman's period is marked as day 1. A woman is fertile about 3-5 days before ovulation and up to 24 hours after the egg has been released. Please refer to the diagram below and the following explanation of pregnancy and how it occurs.

Female Reproductive System

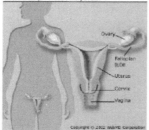

There is mucus that lines the vagina, cervix, and uterus. At the non-fertile times during a woman's cycle, this mucus is very thick and acts as a brick wall for the sperm. At the fertile time during the month, this mucus is very stringy and stretchy. This fertile mucus is necessary for the sperm to survive. When the sperm hits this fertile mucus, the mucus acts as a highway, carrying the sperm through the uterus and fallopian tube where it waits at the end of the fallopian tube for the egg to be released (ovulation). The sperm can last 3-5 days in this fertile mucus, at the end of the fallopian tube. Once ovulation occurs, the fimbrae at the end of the fallopian tube pull the egg in the fallopian tube and fertilization occurs with the meeting of the egg and sperm. This fertilized egg then travels down the fallopian tube to the uterus where it randomly implants into the uterine lining (implantation), it usually takes about 6-10 days from fertilization, for the fertilized egg to travel down and implant.

Once implantation occurs, the hormones begin to change the lining of the uterus to thicken and feed the baby. The hormone hCG is present early during pregnancy and sustains the pregnancy until the development of the placenta where the placenta then maintains the pregnancy through the end. The baby begins to grow rapidly in the first trimester.

Exceptions to the normal cycle rule

Not all women have 28 day cycles or ovulate on day 14, which is an important reason for the ultrasound, to confirm how far along she is according to her last menstrual period (LMP). Her LMP is an estimate, +/- 2 weeks of her estimated date of confinement/due date (EDC). The ultrasound is +/- a few days from her EDC. Therefore, the ultrasound is more accurate in determining how far along she is, vital information for a woman faced with an abortion decision. Knowing how far along she is answers the questions: what procedure will I have and how much it will cost, not to mention the actual fetal development that she sees for that gestation.

Also, for women who have irregular periods, you have to consider the time that her symptoms started and when she thinks conception could have taken place for a more realistic estimate of how far along she is. If a woman has irregular periods, then she is ovulating irregularly as well.

Missed/Belated Period

A patient's menstrual cycle can be interrupted and therefore miss her period or have a belated period for reasons as described below:

1. With any unusual stress or activity, the menstrual cycle can interrupted due to changes in the hormone levels as a direct cause of stress or increase in activity, causing a missed or late period.
2. If she has missed any of her contraceptives or just started something, her body could be getting used to the exposure and she could miss her period or get it late due to the fluctuation in hormone levels. This usually takes a month or two to get on a "normal" schedule which may not be her previous cycle.
3. Some women are so afraid or think they might be pregnant which can induce the hormonal changes causing pregnancy symptoms without a positive pregnancy test.

   A 16 year old in a doctor's office who wanted to be pregnant and thought she was 6 months pregnant related to her LMP. Her pregnancy test was positive, she appeared to have an increase in size of her uterus on palpation, and she was excreting milk form her tender breasts, but when the ultrasound was done, there was no baby in her uterus. The diagnosis was psychological, because she thought she was pregnant and had induced pregnancy symptoms for six months.
4. She could also have a metabolic/Ob/GYN issue going on that needs medical evaluation:
   - ovarian cyst
   - uterine cyst

No matter what the cause, we can tell the patient it is not uncommon to miss a period from time to time, but she should definitely get checked by her OB/GYN doctor. Refer her either to her own physician or give her our referral if she does not have one.

The patient should also be rescheduled for a repeat pregnancy test in 2 weeks if she has not gotten her period. It is possible that she ovulated late in her cycle and that she could be very early on her pregnancy. It is possible that the patient would not have the levels of HCG in her urine that would turn a pregnancy test positive today, but would in 2 weeks, indicating a very early pregnancy.

Contraceptives

Statistics from the Alan Guttmacher Institute (AGI):
- 49% of pregnancies are unintended;
- Almost ½ of unintended pregnancies are ended by an abortion.
- 54 % of women having abortions used a contraceptive during the month they became pregnant.

The data is taken from "Induced Abortion, Facts in Brief" by the Alan Guttmacher Institute and are most current available. Most are from research conducted by AGI. A non-profit Corporation, the research arm of Planned Parenthood.

Hormonal Contraceptives: This category includes birth control pills, the patch, shots and the ring. The morning after pill/Plan B works this way as well.

How they work:

Hormonal Contraceptives work in several different ways to prevent pregnancy
1. Thicken the mucus at the cervix, acting as a brick wall instead of a highway- this does two things, it does not allow the sperm to travel as fast up to the end of the fallopian tube & it does not allow a fertilized egg to travel as fast as it needs to implant into the uterus before menstruation (the sloughing off of the outer most layer of the uterine lining)
2. Prevent or delay ovulation
3. Change the lining in the uterus so that a fertilized egg would not be able to implant

Hormonal Contraceptives do not protect against STD's. They actually increase the risk of STD's for multiple reasons:
1. They alter the female genital tract, increasing a woman's risk of contracting Chlamydia (a bacterial STD) and HIV by 30%. Michael Specter, "AIDS Infection and Birth Control Pills," The Washington Post. June 2, 1987
2. Young women using hormonal contraceptives are thinking about preventing pregnancy and don't realize they are not helping against STD's.
3. They might think that they are protected and have sex more often, therefore increasing their exposure and risk for STD.

How effective they are:

There is perfect use and there is typical use, when talking about effectiveness, as noted below. The perfect use is following the directions exactly as written and not ever being late or missing a pill. Younger people tend to have even worse results than the typical numbers reported.

Hormonal contraceptives are 99% effective with perfect use and about 95% effective with typical use. Young woman can fall into a smaller effectiveness rate (less than 95%) because they are not quite established in their menstrual cycle and their hormone levels are easily disrupted with stress and physical activity, and because they are more likely to forget or miss a pill.

The birth control pills (bcp's) also have different effectiveness for the kind that they are taking. A progesterone only pill is less effective in preventing pregnancy whereas, a combination pill with estrogen is most effective in preventing pregnancy. There are also different types of hormonal contraceptives, the BCP's are the largest category, but other hormonal contraceptive methods include:

1. Patch: use once a week, change it at the beginning of the week. Not as effective as the pill, but you don't have to remember it everyday.
2. Nuva-ring: like a little rubber ring, place it in the vagina and leave it in for three weeks, This method has questionable effectiveness related to other methods.
3. Depo shot: Given in the doctor's office every 13 weeks, can lead to irregular periods, but is most effective in preventing pregnancy in this category.

Barrier Methods: This category includes condoms (both male and female), diaphragm, and cervical caps.

How they work:

Barrier methods work exactly how their name says; they create a barrier of some sort to prevent the sperm from passing through.

How effective they are:

The statistics students are hearing today are for perfect use, but are still fabricated to make condoms look safe and effective. Students are being told that if they use condoms, they are 98-99% effective. The effectiveness of condoms with typical use averages 20% for pregnancy. The only problem is that the teens and young adults we see are actually averaging higher failure rates, than even the typical use as above. These numbers represent failure, which means a woman became pregnant while using condoms. A woman can only get pregnant, is only fertile, one week each month (as discussed in the section previous) So how much more are they not working and we don't realize it because she's not fertile during the rest of the month. Also to keep in mind that STD's are caused by bacteria and viruses that are much smaller than sperm- AND can get through every day.

The FDA reports a failure rate of only 11%, but is only reported in conjunction with PlanB use.

Abstinence is the only 100% effective way to prevent pregnancy and STD's. There are no games that need to be played to prove it! Using these facts allows patients to make informed decisions about their reproductive health.

Below is a chart that demonstrates the difference between the perfect use and typical use of the two most common contraceptives we see our patients use:

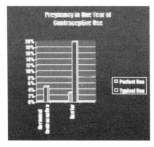

Chart adapted from: Hatcher RA et al, eds., *Contraceptive Technology*, 17th rev. ed., New York: Ardent Media, 1998, Table 9-2, p. 216

Normal Pregnancy Symptoms

"The Top Ten"

1. Abdominal Pain or cramping: this will typically come in the form of menstrual cramping. Some women do not get menstrual cramps, others will report the cramping/pain they are having as unusual. It is important to note if the pain is constant or intermittent and what it feels like. Is it sharp shooting pain? Where is the pain? You want to be concerned if your patient is complaining of pain centered on one side of the abdomen or if they are having constant pain/cramping that does not go away, or is it accompanied by a fever. These could indicate either ectopic pregnancy or miscarriage and should be addressed by their doctor or the ED immediately. They also do not qualify for the ultrasound that you do. The ultrasound is to confirm the viability of the pregnancy. If you do not suspect a viable pregnancy (i.e. ectopic or miscarriage) you will not do an ultrasound.

2. Some light spotting around the time that they would have gotten their period. This usually indicates some implantation bleeding and is not abnormal. Be sure to qualify how much bleeding she had, when she had it, and what color it was. Bright red blood of any amount can be cause for concern. Brown discharge/blood can indicate an old bleed that has finally worked itself out. Be sure to indicate to the patient that if she has any bleeding or spotting, even a pink spot on the toilet paper, she needs to call her doctor or report to the emergency room right away, it could indicate a serious complication and needs to be evaluated.

3. Increase in normal vaginal discharge related to the hormonal changes. Be sure to screen for any discoloration +/or odor as this could indicate an infection and would be a good time to talk about STD testing if either of these are present.

4. Increase in frequency of urination, related to anatomic position of uterus and bladder. As the uterus grows, it decreases the capacity of the bladder causing an increase in urination. They need to be encouraged to continue to maintain their fluid intake and this goes away as the uterus moves up out of the pelvis into the abdomen, usually towards the end of the first trimester. The frequency will return at the end of the third trimester due to the baby settling down into the pelvic area to get ready for delivery. Be sure to screen her for any pain or burning on urination that could indicate a urinary tract infection (UTI). UTI's are very common during pregnancy and since increase in frequency is usually a first sign of a UTI and also a normal finding during pregnancy, we need to be on the look out for further signs and symptoms.

5. Nausea +/or vomiting related to the increase in the hormone levels. This can be happening anytime during the day, *not just in the morning*. The important thing to pass onto patients is that this does not last forever, usually for about 6 weeks from the onset of symptoms. It is also important, as it can be a deciding factor for their situation, that you indicate there are medications that her OB/GYN can prescribe that would help with this problem. Be sure to screen for any hyperemesis where she is not able to keep anything down, this needs medical attention and probable intervention. You could recommend that she eat small meals throughout the day, with crackers in the morning and crackers at bedtime. Also, fresh fruits and fresh vegetables can sometimes curb nausea. The theory behind this is to keep something in the stomach at all times, recognizing that sometimes no matter the intervention, she is still going to have nausea and vomiting. Prenatal vitamins can also induce some nausea as well. Education here could include alternating the time she takes them, maybe at night or with food.

6. Breast tenderness related to an increase in the hormones causing stimulation for breast cell to multiply, with the breasts getting larger during pregnancy. This comes in waves throughout the pregnancy and will be more noticeable for some than others. This is a great introduction for the link between abortion and breast cancer (See the information included).

7. Fatigue is common during early pregnancy. You can encourage her that she will "wake up" into the second trimester.

8. Increased sensitivity to odors: this could be related to the rapid increase in the hormones throughout the body.

9. Food aversions: this may come and go or last throughout the pregnancy.

10. Substance aversions: some women complain that they can't even smoke a whole cigarette for fear they will get sick, or drink alcohol. Call it God's way of telling her it's not healthy, or safe, but it is definitely one way to shake the habits during pregnancy.

Breast Cancer Link to Abortion

The explanation for the link is two fold and multi-dimensional. Recognizing that it is controversial, you need to present the facts and allow them to make a decision based on the facts.

1. Non-controversial link between abortion and breast cancer: It is well known and uncontested that a full term pregnancy alone can decrease a woman's risk of breast cancer. If for no other reason than this, that abortion prevents the protectiveness of a full term pregnancy towards decreasing her risk of breast cancer, a patient who has an abortion is at a higher risk.
2. Controversial link: This is widely known and disputed between the different sides on the abortion issue. It is necessary to present the link stating that it is controversial, but we want them to know, especially if the patient has a history of breast cancer in her family.

The patients need to be told of the link when they are in the office. Brochures are available at abortionbreastcancer.com.

Visiting this website and researching the Abortion Breast Cancer (ABC) Link is on your implementation checklist for this training session.

Script for Breast Cancer link to abortion in patient appointment:

After asking if she has any family history of breast cancer, proceed with the following:

If she has a family history:
"Having a family history of breast cancer, you have an increased risk of breast cancer. Having an abortion could increase that risk further because… " (proceed to below)

If she does not have a family history:
"Having an abortion can increase your risk of breast cancer. Before your first full term pregnancy, your breast cells are what we call Type 1 and Type 2 lobules, or immature breast cells. After 32 weeks of pregnancy, those lobules mature to Type 3 and 4 breast cells. Early during the pregnancy, these Type 1 and 2 lobules begin to multiply as related to the increase in hormones. (as manifested by her tender breasts, and maybe increase in size, draw a graph). After 32 weeks, these multiplied cells mature. This is important because the place where the pre-cancerous cells most often occur is in the Type 1 and Type 2 lobules. Having an abortion, ending a pregnancy before 32 weeks, only increases the number of breast cells vulnerable to the pre-cancerous cells, therefore increasing your risk. It is important for me to note that not every woman who has an abortion will get breast cancer, and not every woman who has breast cancer has had an abortion."

"Do you have any questions related to that information? Does it make sense to you?"

Please have brochures on hand from the above website that gives more information if she seems interested.

Substance use/abuse during pregnancy

1. **Medications:** Ask if she has taken any prescribed or OTC medications. Document which ones, how often and for what. If they are prescription, ask if the prescribing doctor knows that she is pregnant. Encourage her to check with her doctor for the safety of the medications she is taking and a safe plan for stopping if they are not safe during pregnancy. You also want to document why she is taking medications, OTC ones to be sure she doesn't need medical attention for a specific problem and Prescription, just to know what her health history is and see if any of the conditions she has may be of concern for her as related to her pregnancy.

Remember that you are not her medical provider and it is very important that she seek his/her input for her medications as the benefits to her taking them may outweigh the risks to her pregnancy. You also don't want to concern her or give her any additional reason to think she should not carry her pregnancy to term by giving information regarding risks of medications specific to her. Only say, "I do not know if the medications you are taking are recommended during pregnancy. You should check with your doctor to be sure." You can tell her OTC things like Ibuprofen are not recommended and she should only take Tylenol or acetaminophen for headaches, etc.

2. **Drugs:** Ask if she is taking any street drugs and educate her that they are not recommended during pregnancy. Marijuana is the only drug I have run up against at CompassCare and it is related to babies small for gestational age and preterm delivery. Obviously some drugs can cause withdrawal for the baby and lead to other complications. Be sure whatever you say to her is approved by your Medical Director.

3. **Smoking:** You want to know how much she smoked before she found out she is pregnant. Most of the time she will automatically decrease smoking even though she may not be intending on keeping her pregnancy, this is something you can use to encourage her—that she is doing a great job and that it sounds like she cares about what happens during her pregnancy. Smoking can also lead to small for gestational age and preterm delivery. You should educate her that it is not recommended that she smoke during her pregnancy, praise out the positive steps she is taking towards quitting, and encourage her to seek her OB/GYN's help in quitting if she has any problems.

4. **Alcohol:** Ask if she has drank, how often, what and how much. Document all of these in the space provided and encourage her that drinking is not recommended during pregnancy. This may be an area where she is very concerned about her baby, and any damage that may have been done. You can say that it sounds like she is concerned about her baby and reassure her that stopping now definitely decreases any risk to her baby. Also encourage her that if she is still early, she may not have had much, if any exposure, we'll have to wait and see what the ultrasound shows.

At any time when talking to her about the above issues, do not be judgmental. Do not condemn her for the decisions she has made, but encourage her for the concern she has and keep this interaction professional and positive.

Documentation of OB history and current care

As liability is a huge issue for the Pregnancy Resource Center, this is one area we can not leave blank. It is necessary to identify who she will be seeking care from. If she does not have anybody, she will need to be referred. Through medical follow-up, this issue must be addressed until you have a name of her MD documented.

It is important to note, as you will in the Ultrasound consent, that follow-up care is not provided. If she has any questions or concerns related to her pregnancy care or symptoms, she should always be directed back to her own doctor. If she has any general questions, she should have access to ask you, but know that they should be referred to her doctor.

130

Sexual History

Ask how many sexual partners she has had and look at the "How at risk are you?" brochure that has the chart of sexual exposure in it. Point out where she is now in terms of the number of sexual partners she has had. Where does she want to be when she gets married? Where does she want her husband to be? Does she want to get married? What does that mean for her? What does she value in a relationship? What is important to her (communication, friendship...)? Where does sex fit in? Challenge her to make decisions based on her own values that you have just discussed.

Ask the patient how she plans on preventing pregnancy in the future.

Ask the patient if she thought about not having sex until she got married. Would that be possible for her? Talk about how that would change their relationship. What would that look like? How could she continue her present relationship? What would she say/do with her boyfriend that would promote that decision? Is she willing to lose her boyfriend if he doesn't agree with her new decision? Give her "Sex, Been there, Done that, Now What" brochure so she can read that and get creative in her decision making.

Empower her to stand up for her beliefs and values. Capitalize on her strengths, enabling her to make these decisions outside of your office.

This is a great place to do some minor education on STD's, and to present and offer of the STD testing at your center.

Rochester is #1 and #2 in the nation for Gonorrhea and Chlamydia. They are bacterial STD's that are treatable and curable if you know you have it. Up to 80% of people who have them do not have symptoms, the majority of them being women. All of our patients who have tested positive have had no idea.

STD's and Pregnancy:
It is a great place to note that if she does have Chlamydia or Gonorrhea at this time, her pregnancy is protecting her from it spreading. She has a mucus plug in her cervix which is at the end of her vagina, opening into the uterus. This plug will not allow that bacteria to pass through, it is trapped in the vaginal canal. Some STD's are able to get into the blood stream and cause problems with the pregnancy and fetal development. The other good news is that it is easily treatable during pregnancy and is curable. Another great thing about these two infections, specifically, is that they do not get into the blood stream and can cause little if any harm to the pregnancy. The viral STD's are the ones that pass through and the two most concerning are Herpes and HIV. A woman will be tested for STD's at her prenatal physical and will be followed up appropriately by her OB/GYN.

STD's and Abortion:
> Of patients who have a Chlamydia infection at the time of their abortion, 25% will develop PID within 4 weeks.

During an abortion, the bacteria can be introduced and forced into the uterus where the lining has just been irritated form the procedure. This is an environment where the bacteria can grow and the STD can spread through the entire reproductive system, causing life-long damage.

PID: Pelvic Inflammatory Disease is the advanced stages of Gonorrhea and Chlamydia

PID can cause infertility and an increase risk of ectopic pregnancy.
Infertility- the inability to have children
Ectopic Pregnancy- a life-threatening pregnancy in the tubes

Women should be tested for STD's whether they have been with the same person for years. Education on routine visits to OB/GYN for Pap tests and STD testing for her reproductive health should also take place at this time.

PLEASE NOTE: This is not the time to preach about abstinence. This is a time to ease her most pressing fears and begin a relationship that will facilitate the making of good decisions and feed into the importance of every decision she makes as she is followed up with throughout her pregnancy.

Any other medical conditions/treatments

This is a great question to ask and essential to not be skipped for any reason. This is the opportunity she has to express any other concerns she has in carrying her pregnancy to term from a medical stand point. The most often responses you will hear are chronic conditions (i.e. back pain, cysts on ovaries or uterus, bleeding disorders, etc.) or that the patient will specifically say that she was told she should never have children because of.... This is where you will either give her peace by directly responding to the issue or let her know that you will find out, by asking your medical director, and get back to her when you confirm her pregnancy. You want to be careful not to discredit any provider she has had in the past, therefore losing any report you may have with her. You also don't want to guess at a response—you are not her medical provider and even though you have just completed the Health History with her, you still don't know everything about her.

23. Confidentiality Policy and Procedure

Confidentiality occurs when there is an exchange of information made in trust between individuals or groups with the overt understanding that none of the information will be given to any other individual, group, or entity without the written consent of the patient.

PROCEDURE:

1. All patients will be protected from disclosure of information that violates their right to privacy except where required by law, i.e. child abuse, suicide prevention… Professional ethics require responsibility for maintaining the confidentiality of private information.

2. CPS personnel shall be responsible for maintaining the confidentiality of private information. Disclosure by and between volunteers/employees of private information shall occur only as necessary to carry out job functions.

3. Information shall be released to third parties only upon written authorization from the patient. An Authorization to Release Records Form must be signed by the patient. The written authorization will be time limited and not exceed 90 days from the date of signature. The written authorization will be witnessed by a staff person or volunteer of the office.

4. No confidential information will be released to anyone, even the patient, over the telephone.

5. If questioned about a patient's records and there is no existing written authorization, the correct response is, "Due to confidentiality, I cannot verify the client has ever been seen or treated at the office, nor can I tell you that the requested records are on file." The patient can then be contacted by the office staff to let her know a request for records was made and the patient can determine if she would like to provide a written authorization to release the information to the party making the request.

References

2011 Florida Statutes 766.103.3(a)1. Florida Medical Consent Law. 2011 [cited 31 Oct 2011]. Available from: http://www.leg. state.fl.us/Statutes/

Abram, Morris B. (Chairman, President's Commission for the Study of Ethical Problems in Medicine and Biomedical and Behavioral Research). Letter to: The President. 21 Oct 1982 [cited 9 Sep 2011]. 1 leaf. Printed in: Making Health Care Decisions: The Ethical and Legal Implications of Informed Consent in the Patient-Practitioner Relationship. Vol. 1. Washington: GPO; 1982.

American College of Obstetricians and Gynecologists. The limits of conscientious refusal in reproductive medicine. ACOG Committee Opinion No. 385. *Obstet Gynecol.* 2007;110(5):1203-8.

American College of Physicians. *Ethics Manual.* 4th ed. *Ann Intern Med.* 1998;128(7):576-94.

Andrew LB. Expert witness testimony: The ethics of being a medical expert witness. *Emerg Med Clin North Am.* 2006; 24(3):715-31.

Aristotle. *Metaphysics.* Trans. Ross WD. 1.1.7 [cited 11 Apr 2011]. Available from: http://classics.mit.edu/Aristotle/metaphysics.1.i.html (981b27-30).

Barbacci MB, Spence M, Kappus EW, Murkman RC, Rao L, Quinn TC. Postabortal endometritis and isolation of Chlamydia trachomatis. *Obstet Gynecol.* 1986;68(5):686-90.

Beauchamp TL, Childress JF. *Principles of Biomedical Ethics.* 6th ed. New York: Oxford University Press; 2009.

Chacko MR, Lovchik JC. Chiamydia trachomatis infection in sexually active adolescents: Prevalence and risk factors. *Pediatrics*. 1984;73(6):836-40.

Daling JR, Malone KE, Voigt LF, White E, Weiss NS. Risk of breast cancer among young women: Relationship to induced abortion. *J Natl Cancer Inst*. 1994;86(21):1584-92.

Declaration of Independence of the United States, 1776.

Duthie SJ, Hobson D, Tait IA, Pratt BC, Lowe N, Sequeira PJ, et al. Morbidity after termination of pregnancy in first trimester. *Genitourin Med*. 1987;63(3):182-7.

Finer LB, Frohwirth LF, Dauphinee LA, Singh S, Moore AM. Guttmacher Institute. Reasons U.S. women have abortions: Quantitative and qualitative perspectives. *Perspect Sex Reprod Health*. 2005;37(3):110-8.

Friedenwald H. The ethics of the practice of medicine from the Jewish point of view. Bulletin of the John Hopkins Hospital. 1917;28(318):255-61.

General Assembly of the United Nations. Universal Declaration of Human Rights. 1948.

van den Heever P. Pleading the defense of therapeutic privilege. *S Afr Med J*. 2005;95(6):420-1.

Hippocrates. *The Hippocratic Oath*. Trans. in Kass LR. *Toward a More Natural Science*. New York: Simon and Schuster; 1988:228-9.

Hippocrates. *The Hippocratic Oath*. Trans. North M. National Library of Medicine; 2002 [cited 11 Apr 2011]. Available from: http://www.nlm.nih.gov/hmd/greek/greek_oath.html

Lasagna L. A Modern Hippocratic Oath. 1964 [cited 3 Aug 2011]. Available from: http://www.aapsonline.org/ethics/oaths.htm#lasagna

National Abortion Federation. 2011 Clinical Policy Guidelines.

Washington: National Abortion Federation; 2011.

Orr, RD. Critique of ACOG Committee Opinion #385, November 2007. Christian Medical and Dental Association. 2008 [cited 2 Nov 2011]. Available from: http://www.cmda. org/WCM/CMDA/Issues2/Healthcare1/Conscience_Rights/ Articles_and_Commentaries6/CMDA_ Member_s_Commen. aspx

Ovigstad E, Skaug K, Jerve F, Fylling P, Ulstrup JC. Pelvic inflammatory disease associated with Chlamydia trachomatis infection after therapeutic abortion: A prospective study. *Br J Vener Dis*. 1983;59(3):189-92.

Percival T. Medical Ethics; Or a Code of Institutes and Precepts Adapted to the Professional Conduct of Physicians and Surgeons. Manchester: S. Russell; 1803.

President's Commission for the Study of Ethical Problems in Medicine and Biomedical and Behavioral Research. Making Health Care Decisions: The Ethical and Legal Implications of Informed Consent in the Patient-Practitioner Relationship. Vol. 1. Washington: GPO; 1982.

Rasinski KA, Yoon JD, Kalad YG, Curlin FA. Obstetrician-gynaecologists' opinions about conscientious refusal of a request for abortion: results from a national vignette experiment. *J Med Ethics*. Published online 13 Jun 2011 [cited 2 Nov 2011]. Available from: http://jme. bmj.com/content/early/2011/06/13/jme.201 0.040782. abstract?sid=306877bb-775d-4c9b-bdcc- 30acbab50b92

Rooney B, Calhoun BC. Induced abortion and risk of later premature births. *J Am Phys Surg*. 2003;8(2):46-9.

Rue VM, Coleman PK, Rue JJ, Reardon DC. Induced abortion and traumatic stress: A preliminary comparison of American and Russian women. *Med Sci Monit*. 2004;10(10):SR5-16.

Southard P, Frankel P. Trauma care documentation: A comprehensive guide. *J Emerg Nurs.* 1989;15(5):393-8.

Stewart MA. Effective physician-patient communication and health outcomes: A review. *Can Med Assoc J.* 1995;152(9):1423- 33.

Utah Code 78B-3-406.1(f). Chapter 3, 2008 General Session; 2008 [cited 31 Oct 2011]. Available from: http://le.utah.gov/ Documents/code_const.htm.

Wear, S. Ethics Committee Core Curriculum: Informed Consent. UB Center for Clinical Ethics and Humanities in Health Care, University of Buffalo; 2006 [cited 31 Oct 2011]. Available from: http://wings.buffalo.edu/bioethics/man-infc. html.

Westergaard L, Philipsen T, Scheibel J. Significance of cervical Chlamydia trachomatis infection in postabortal pelvic infla\ matory disease. *Obstet Gynecol.* 1982;60(3):322-5.